# START WHERE YOU ARE

# START WHERE YOU ARE

## THE BEGINNER'S 5K RUNNING GUIDE FOR WOMEN

### SABRINA PACE-HUMPHREYS

BLOOMSBURY SPORT
LONDON · OXFORD · NEW YORK · NEW DELHI · SYDNEY

BLOOMSBURY SPORT
Bloomsbury Publishing Plc
50 Bedford Square, London, WC1B 3DP, UK
29 Earlsfort Terrace, Dublin 2, Ireland

BLOOMSBURY, BLOOMSBURY SPORT and the
Diana logo are trademarks of Bloomsbury Publishing Plc

First published in Great Britain 2026
Text copyright © Sabrina Pace-Humphreys, 2026
Author photograph © Tanya Raab, 2026

Sabrina Pace-Humphreys has asserted her right under the Copyright,
Designs and Patents Act, 1988, to be identified as Author of this work.

For legal purposes the Acknowledgements on p. 250 constitute an extension of this copyright page

All rights reserved. No part of this publication may be: i) reproduced or transmitted in any form, electronic or mechanical, including photocopying, recording or by means of any information storage or retrieval system without prior permission in writing from the publishers; or ii) used or reproduced in any way for the training, development or operation of artificial intelligence (AI) technologies, including generative AI technologies. The rights holders expressly reserve this publication from the text and data mining exception as per Article 4(3) of the Digital Single Market Directive (EU) 2019/790

Bloomsbury Publishing Plc does not have any control over, or responsibility for, any third-party websites referred to or in this book. All internet addresses given in this book were correct at the time of going to press. The author and publisher regret any inconvenience caused if addresses have changed or sites have ceased to exist, but can accept no responsibility for any such changes

A catalogue record for this book is available from the British Library

Library of Congress Cataloguing-in-Publication data has been applied for

The information contained in this book is provided by way of general guidance in relation to the specific subject matters addressed herein, but it is not a substitute for specialist advice. It should not be relied on for medical, health-care, pharmaceutical or other professional advice on specific dietary or health needs. This book is sold with the understanding that the author and publisher are not engaged in rendering medical, health or any other kind of personal or professional services. The reader should consult a competent medical or health professional before adopting any of the suggestions in this book or drawing inferences from it. The author and publisher specifically disclaim, as far as the law allows, any responsibility from any liability, loss or risk (personal or otherwise) which is incurred as a consequence, directly or indirectly, of the use and applications of any of the contents of this book.

ISBN: TPB: 978-1-3994-2331-1; ePUB: 978-1-3994-2332-8; ePDF: 978-1-3994-2330-4

2 4 6 8 10 9 7 5 3 1

Typeset in IBM Plex Serif by Lumina Datamatics Ltd
Printed and bound in Great Britain by Clays Ltd, Elcograf S.p.A.

To find out more about our authors and books visit www.bloomsbury.com
and sign up for our newsletters

For product safety related questions contact productsafety@bloomsbury.com

# Contents

| | |
|---|---|
| 1: I don't DO running | 6 |
| 2: You ARE a runner | 13 |
| 3: Don't sweat the technique | 25 |
| 4: Gearing up to run | 40 |
| 5: All the feels | 63 |
| 6: Walk this way | 76 |
| 7: Mounds of opportunity | 87 |
| 8: Safety matters | 106 |
| 9: Don't stop, period! | 122 |
| 10: Menopause matters | 138 |
| 11: Stronger than yesterday | 160 |
| 12: You get out what you put in | 195 |
| 13: Miles and smiles | 212 |
| 14: A final message from me . . . | 244 |
| References | 246 |
| Bibliography | 249 |
| Acknowledgements | 250 |
| Index | 252 |

CHAPTER 1

# I don't DO running

When it comes to learning to run, I have been where you are right now, and I remember it like it was yesterday.

It was a late summer's day in 2009 when I made the decision to 'try to run'. I remember every single emotion, every feeling of fear and trepidation. And I can still viscerally feel that bubble of anxiety that grew so big inside me that it almost stopped me even stepping out of the door.

Back then I didn't know a thing about running and, if I am being honest, I felt too embarrassed to ask. Why? Because I was worried that people might laugh at me for even daring to try. You see, I didn't look like a runner, I didn't act like a runner, and I didn't know any women who I could relate to who ran. It didn't feel like running was for someone like me.

**REASONS YOU MIGHT TAKE UP RUNNING**

- Time for yourself
- Stress relief
- To feel stronger
- To strengthen your bones
- To deal with the effects of ageing
- To manage symptoms of the perimenopause/menopause
- Connection with others
- To challenging yourself
- Mental health management
- Weight management

In those early days, I needed the woman I am now as my cheerleader. The female runner I have grown to be. A person who with empathy, lived experience, knowledge and expertise could show me the way. Could answer every question I had.

I needed the book you are about to read.

This book is going to tell you everything you need to know to go from the couch to 5K (C25K) in 10 weeks. It contains background information that other running books just don't. And what makes it even more special – and badly needed – is that it's aimed specifically at you: a *woman* at the start of her journey!

Do you want to know how to integrate running into your life, so it becomes a habit? That's on p. 21. Worried about your safety while running – I've got you! See chapter 8. Anxious about running while on your period? See chapter 9. Need some gear but have no idea? I'll share my essentials with you in chapter 4.

I've crammed as much information on all aspects of learning to run into this book as I possibly can. I have shared my own expertise and experience and have also sought advice from other experts and many female runners who were once exactly where you are now.

It's all here in this book. Waiting for you.

### MY 5K AND ME

'I signed up to join a women-only C25K group and, on my way there, felt so anxious that I turned back. What the hell was I thinking? Another woman was walking towards me and asked if I was joining the new group. I muttered "Yes" and she said she'd walk with me, as she was joining, too. I went to that session and realised that there were other women of all shapes and sizes who wanted to learn to run, just like me. And that inclusiveness felt good. I never missed a session and completed my first 5K feeling amazing. I am now a run leader with that group!'

## Use it, don't lose it

My first piece of advice to you is to *read this book before you start* the 10-week running plan I have designed for you in the Miles and Smiles chapter on page 212. Use this book as a journal. Write questions in the margins, scribble down thoughts and contact me on social media. Read this book through once, twice if you want to. But, please, *do* read it before you start running.

Experience has shown me that to be forewarned is to be forearmed, so reading this book first will ensure you have all the advice and tools you need to ensure your running practice goes well.

## Trust in me?!

Before we get into the nitty-gritty there are a few things I feel you need to know about me: why I do what I do and why I have written this book. A few things that will, I hope, strengthen your bond and trust in me.

First and foremost, I am a qualified UK Athletics Run Leader and Run Coach. I am also a qualified personal trainer. And, of course, I am a runner.

I am also a 47-year-old mother of four and grandmother of three.

Since 2016 I have coached many women, both in person and online, to learn to run distances from 5K to ultramarathon (distances greater than 42.2km/26.2 miles). I have volunteered my coaching services at formal athletics clubs and, in 2016, I founded a women-only running community in my local town: Stroud Mums on the Run. I am proud to still lead this community today.

I am passionate about using running to promote mental and physical wellness and, in 2024, I was awarded an honorary doctorate for my achievements – running being the conduit for many of these. Talking about the power of running and its ability to change lives is one of my favourite things to do.

But I wasn't always a runner...

## Postnatal depression

I started running in 2009 on advice from my GP following the birth of my fourth child. A diagnosis of postnatal depression led to the GP suggesting some things that, alongside medication and talk therapy, might help manage my illness. To 'try a jog' was one of them. I had never run before. I did not know anyone who ran and, at that time, I was about 32kg (5 stone) overweight. It took me days to get out of the door because I was anxious but, in the end, I was willing to try anything to feel mentally better and said to myself, 'If a GP tells you to try it, how bad can it be?' I found a quiet spot and shuffled my wobbly, shaky body for a mile (this was too far but back then I didn't know any better). Everything hurt. Bits of me I'd never felt before hurt. When I finished, I fell in the door. But once I'd dragged myself to the shower I realised that, during the shuffle, there had been one thing that was less intrusive – my dark thoughts. I knew that I wanted to feel that sense of relief again; that's what helped me go out again and again and again.

> **SOCIAL PRESCRIBING**
>
> Social prescribing is where a healthcare professional will refer you to non-medical activities and services to improve your well-being, such as gym classes, art, meditation, gardening and running. Since 2023, at least 25 countries have introduced social prescribing.

## A new identity

I didn't know it then, on that run in 2009, that running would change my life as I knew it. I don't use the words 'running changed my life' lightly. I'm not one to play with words; they have power. But it did. Something happened to me that day. A freedom. A glimmer of hope. An escape. The act of running seeped into my system: like a vaccination through a needle, it seeped into my bloodstream, my body, my brain, taking hold of something inside me like a drug and – even though, MY LORD!, it was so very hard in those early days – and on many, many days since – I wanted to try again. I needed to try again. For me. For my children. I wanted to try again, and again, and again. Until maybe it didn't seem so hard.

For a year I practised my running alone. But, as well as for my mental health, I wanted to run 'for something' like a small distance, so I chose 5km (3.1 miles; often called 5K, which is how I like to style distances). In those days there were no free weekly 5K Parkruns. There were no female-only running groups (well, not that I could find in my area anyway). The only representation of runners that I saw locally were lithe white men and women who ran in short shorts and vests or crop tops. People who trained and raced each other in packs – like dogs – along the roads and hills (yes, they raced each other up hills – crazy!). They donned the same-colour vests and T-shirts like it was their special uniform. And that green they wore would never look good on someone like me anyway . . .

Their demeanour, their speed and their attire subconsciously yelled, '*This* is what a runner looks like and, if you don't look like this – thin, fast, like us – then you don't fit in. You are not a runner.'

> **WHAT IS PARKRUN?**
>
> Parkrun is a free community event at which you can walk, jog, run, volunteer or spectate. It is 5km (3.1 miles) in distance and takes place every Saturday morning.

## Breaking down barriers

I've been running for more than 15 years now – a touch under a third of my life. I have dedicated, willingly, hours and hours of time to practising running. I like to use simple terms for what I do weekly because using terminology that feels threatening, that feels as though you need a degree in sports science to understand, is a barrier to women accessing this activity. And anyone who know me knows I'm all about breaking down barriers.

So, yes, I have spent hours *practising* my running. Just like other people practise mindfulness or yoga, I practise running. And that practice has led me to set goals for myself that enabled me to run for longer and longer. My practice led to me setting a goal to run 5K (3.1 miles) in 2009 and to go on, over the years, to complete 10K (6.2 miles), my first ever half marathon (22.1km/13.1 miles) in 2010 and my first ever marathon (42.2km/26.2 miles) in 2011 – making me one of the 0.01 per cent of the global population to have completed that distance – and in 2022 I ran my longest ultramarathon to date – 268 miles along the UK's oldest footpath – The Pennine Way.

The self-belief and understanding that I have acquired through my running practice, through my own goal-setting, has been life-changing. Having the confidence to enquire about and join a running club where there was a group for slower runners resulted in me meeting other women who felt as anxious as I did, who felt as out of place as I did, who didn't understand the terminology either, but who wanted to practise with others like them, too. It felt like a gift.

Because making the commitment to try running can be scary. It can feel threatening as a woman. It can make you ask yourself, 'Do I belong here?' It can make others question your decision to practise running and even describe you as selfish for taking time to do it.

But I'm here to call bullshit on that. I challenge that narrative daily. Why?

Because running as a tool to help manage the stresses and strains of life matters. Because running has enabled me, and many other women I know, to reclaim a sense of themselves. To find deep wells of physical and mental strength and resilience that we didn't know we possessed. To find friendship in the common practice of this activity. To be the representation that they, and others, needed to see.

To find community. To find safety. To find sisterhood.

To claim the mantle of 'runner'.

## Finding strength in community

When I find something that works for me, I want to share it with everyone – to the point that I know I can be annoying. But I make no apologies for that. If I find something that I love, I want everyone to feel it. What's the point of finding a secret elixir, the magic medicine, if no one else knows about it?

In 2016, when I qualified as a UK Athletics Run Leader, I decided to launch a women-only run group in my local town. Thirty brave women turned up on a cold winter's day feeling that same trepidation and fear that I did in 2009, wondering whether they could 'do it'. Thinking, in many cases, that they couldn't.

I worked with them over the course of 10 weeks to show them – through well-planned practice, through online support and the solidarity they found in being part of my community, through ticking off small goals as each week went by – that they could. That they were runners, too. That, although their lives may be different, in this space, they were the same. They experienced the same fears, the same struggles and the same wins. There was strength in community, as women supporting women.

They were safe.

All my women completed that first 5K with me. Some of those women still come out and run with me. And hundreds of women, since 2016, have started their running journey with me. I could not be more grateful to them for choosing me. For continuing to choose me. This virtuous cycle of them giving me what I need as a woman and a run coach and that innate sense of purpose I get when I see them succeeding – and me sharing in that achievement they feel when they reach their goals – is a winning combination.

You are part of that community now, whether you are a brand-new female runner or a woman who is coming back to running after a break.

Throughout these pages, many women around the world have allowed me to share their advice, their tips and their stories with you. They are women who have been in the same place as you are right now.

I am going to take you on a literal, mental, physical and joyful – yes, it *will* be joyful – journey. I am going to share with you everything I believe you need to know to learn – over a 5K journey – to run safe, run strong and run free as a woman.

I want you to have all of the information you need to succeed. The running sisterhood wants to share this with you.

So, are you ready to start from where you are?

Let's go.

Small steps, big change.

## CHAPTER 2

# You ARE a runner

How did it make you feel when I referred to you as a runner in the previous chapter? Did you shudder? Did you laugh out loud? Did you think, 'She's lost the plot, I'm no runner'?

Well, to me, you are a runner. But part of the reason you don't believe it – or can't believe it yet – is because you have been conditioned not to think of yourself like that. Because you might feel anxious that people – whoever they are – might think you're too big for your boots, they might think, 'Who the hell does she think she is?!'

There's a ton of research out there that shows that men will often exhibit higher confidence in their athletic abilities compared to women. If I was asking a man to think of themselves as a runner, as a recreational athlete, they would likely claim that mantle far more quickly than you feel comfortable to. It's the conditioning.

When you hear the word 'runner' or even 'athlete', who do you think of? Is it the name of an elite sportswoman, an Olympian, that comes to mind? If so, you are not alone. It's those women who, throughout our lives, we've been conditioned to associate with those words. It isn't Pam next door.

But I'm here to explain a simple truth: YOU are a runner, too. Even if only, right now, in mind.

And mindset is everything.

I was watching something on TV the other day and it reinforced to me, once again, why your journey as a runner is so important to me and why this book needed to be written. It was August 2024 and the final day of the Olympics in Paris. I was listening to Dame Laura Kenny, who won numerous medals for Team GB in track cycling, talk about the life of an elite track cyclist. She said that, 'When they are not training or racing, they try *not* to stand up.' Why? Because any energy that they expend by standing up is less energy they have available for their body to recruit when training or racing. She recalled a quote from another retired elite athlete, Sir Chris Hoy: 'Never stand when you can sit, never sit when you can lie down.'

I laughed and thought to myself, 'Ah, the life of an elite athlete.' Because – like many of you – as a woman who works, is a mother, a grandmother, a run coach, PT, author, runner and recreational athlete, I just do not have that privilege. If I can grab an afternoon nap – which sometimes perimenopause (more about that later) demands – then I feel I've had a very lucky day indeed.

Your journey to learn to run needs to work for you and suit the life demands that you have but, because of the additional life stressors that you'll have to deal with, I believe you'll be *even more* resilient than an elite athlete (yes, you!) because you are having to juggle a multitude of other life demands too.

If I could put the gold medal around your neck, I would. Just for even getting to the stage of contemplation that you are at right now.

## Why are you here?

What made you pick up this book, at this time in your life, and start reading it where you are right now?

Because you know there's a reason, right? Maybe your why is . . .

'I want to feel fitter.'

'I want some headspace away from the family.'

'I want to be able to run around after my kids/grandkids.'

'I want to do something just for me.'

'I've been inspired by someone I know; I want to try to learn to run, too.'

There is no such thing as chance. I believe that 'everything happens for a reason'. And, to start with, I want you to challenge the perceptions you have of yourself as a runner. To truly start to claim that word for yourself, there are some stereotypes, barriers and mindset shifts that, with the help of experts, I want to help you understand.

You might feel a bit uncomfortable. And that's OK. Because those feelings of uncomfortableness are part of our journey when starting, and continuing, to run. I'm going to help you to 'get comfortable with being uncomfortable'. Because I truly believe that the greatest change comes from that. From feeling it and moving through to the other side.

But, please always know, I have your physical and mental safety at heart; everything I write about in this book is intended to empower you.

Because knowledge is power. The stories of other women gives power. You are powerful.

You haven't run a step yet, or maybe even put on a pair of trainers, so how can I have the audacity to ask you to believe that you are an athlete, a runner?

Here's why.

## Representation matters

Do you know what stopped me ever thinking that running was for me until I was 31 years old? Here are some of the reasons:

- I didn't see runners who looked like me.
- It looked too hard.
- I didn't know 'how' to run.
- I didn't know where to go that was safe.
- I felt I would be laughed at.
- I didn't know women who experienced some of the same barriers to running that I had.
- I didn't know women who felt the same anxiety when starting to run as I had.

These limiting factors were a problem. They created a barrier to access.

And when I talk about women, I am talking about all intersectionalities of woman – from women of colour to those with invisible illnesses, from fuller-bodied women to women who identify as part of the LGBTQIA+ community, from teenage girls to grandmothers. It's so important that I say this – and I'm going to say it loudly: WE ARE NOT A MONOLITH. What one woman sees as a barrier to them starting, and continuing, to run, may not feel like a barrier for another. This is something I will continue to discuss in this book. But, of course, there are commonalities in the reasons that so many of us feel we can't run.

Here are some of the most common reasons:

- Not feeling safe
- Not finding other women who wanted to learn to run
- Not being fast enough
- Running being 'not for bigger bodies'
- Low self-confidence and self-image
- No idea 'where to start'
- False medical narratives: 'running will give me bad knees'
- Not feeling confidence with sport at school
- Time commitment versus family needs

And the list goes on . . .

## It's not me, it's you

The reason that you might not feel a sense of belonging or that you fit the traditional 'runner' stereotype is not your problem, it's theirs – the people in charge of portraying what constitutes a runner. Often men.

### CASE STUDY 1

In 2020, a running brand wrote a post on what was then Twitter about some 'office banter', which, they stated, might even form part of their employee handbook. For me, and so many others who know all too well what it takes to start running as a woman, this post did not land well.

> The headline was 'How Not to Be a Jogger', and it detailed things that 'you definitely don't want to be caught doing on a run' – things that 'real runners' wouldn't be caught dead doing.
>
> The list included more than 13 of their unwritten rules. All utterly deplorable. All elitist. All damaging. According to them, you are not a 'real runner' if you:
>
> - Wear a jacket around your waist
> - Wear a phone armband
> - Tuck your T-shirt in
> - Jog on the spot if you hit a traffic light
> - Wear a waist belt to hold some food or drink
> - Text while you are running

Have you ever heard anything more ridiculous?!

Lots of us hit back – of course – and the brand backtracked (as they often do when they are caught out). But what they displayed, and what many people in charge of sports marketing display, is the inherent running snobbery problem: that if you don't behave in a certain way, look a certain way, run a certain way – you don't belong.

I want to address these right now.

NO ONE gets to tell you whether you are a runner or not. Not men in suits. Not sports marketers in city firms. Not the next-door neighbour. Not an influencer. If we as female runners allow our experiences, the things that can bring us joy, health and friendship, to be dictated by others, then we will never feel the sense of freedom that I know running can bring us.

- If you run and you are overweight, you are a runner.
- If you run a 20-, or a 30-, 40-, 50- or 60- minute 5K, you are a runner.
- If you run for two minutes, you are a runner.
- If you run with your jumper tied around your waist, you are a runner.
- If you run with a bum bag or backpack, you are a runner.

- If you run holding a bottle of water, you are a runner.
- If you run with the kids while they're on their bikes, you are a runner.
- If you run once a week, you are a runner.
- If you walk during your runs, you are a runner.
- If you start sweating after one minute, you are a runner.
- If you only run in spring, or summer, or winter, you are a runner.

I mean, the list could go on indefinitely, but you catch my drift. These man-made, old-school perceptions have created barriers that we need to take down.

Only 6 per cent of sports-related research is conducted on female-only participants. All of the rest of the studies that inform programmes and products designed to help us learn to run, decide what to wear, how to fuel, how we recover, etc., have historically been done on men. They are not based on our needs as women, our bodies, our minds, our physiology. Dr Stacy Sims – a respected scientist in this field – reminds us that 'women are not small men'. How we respond to running is not the same as how men respond, so why are so many training programmes based on science that isn't for us? That doesn't maximise our hormonal and energy highs and lows to suit our menstrual cycle, perimenopause and menopause.

But don't worry, I've got you – I will go into this, with the help of experts in their field, in later chapters.

When it comes to the perception of what it is to be a female runner it's only in the last few years, with inclusive marketing campaigns such as the This Girl Can campaign here in the UK and the work of an army of female leaders in sport from grassroots to boardroom level, that representation of all intersectionalities of female runners have been seen.

And not only seen but *celebrated*.

Here are just a few of the inspiring female runners we love to see:

- Mirna Valerio
- Jo Pavey

- Kelly Holmes
- Paula Radcliffe
- Courtney Dauwalter
- Sophie Raworth
- Shelly-Ann Fraser-Pryce

## You can't be what you can't see

Be honest with me now, if I asked you what a female runner looked like, what would you say? Here's what – some years ago – I said:

'She's thin. She's muscly. You can see all her muscle definition and her veins popping out of her skin because she's got barely any fat on her, because she runs so much. She's got a ponytail that bounces up and down as she runs. She looks so light and bouncy. She's probably in shorts and a vest top. I'm nothing like her.'

I would have given you that answer because, most of the time, that is what I saw. That is what marketing executives presented to me. That 'woman' was the go-to model of what a female runner looked like. And, if you weren't that, then running might not be such a good place for you to be.

## Failure to launch

I have coached many hundreds of women, and the one thing that holds them back from even trying is the fear of failure. Of 'not being able to do it'. Of not being good enough.

And I tell them the same thing time and time again: 'I have been where you are. You are good enough. Trust me and let me help you find your running joy.'

It takes a shift in mindset to change your thought process around identity and belonging as a runner. And more than that, it takes surrounding yourself with people who challenge your perceptions around what a runner looks like, how a runner moves, what a runner wears and eats and how a runner practises, for you to build confidence.

> **NO WOMAN LEFT BEHIND**
>
> Tasha Thompson, founder of Black Girls Do Run UK, has this to say: *'No woman left behind* is a phrase that is so important to me because we have to remember that we were all beginners once! Each one of us knows how it feels to start running. How it feels like everything hurts all at once and how it's hard to breathe. For me, running is about creating a safe space. If a woman is running with us, they can be guaranteed that I stand by these words in actions and deeds. You will not be left behind! You are safe and you are seen. And it's a phrase that transcends running. In life, we must uplift our sisters. *No woman left behind!'*

## Mind over matter – where are you now?

You know that saying, 'The mind will give way before the body does.' It really is true. I used to think that taking up running was a snap decision that I made but, after that initial consultation with my GP, I started going through a process of change.

Small steps lead to big change. You might not know it, but you have already taken small steps on your journey of change.

A few years ago, I was invited onto a BBC podcast about women and exercise, alongside Dr Candice Lingam-Willgoss, associate dean and senior lecturer for The Open University and a sports scientist. We were talking about mindset when it comes to exercise and creating habits. Candice discussed the five stages of change that people go through when learning any new habit. The change model is called the Transtheoretical Model of Behaviour. When it comes to your running journey, it looks a bit like this:

## THE FIVE STAGES OF BEGINNER RUNNING BEHAVIOUR

1. *Nope. No way I am a runner, not even thinking about it* (pre-contemplation – not ready stage)
   For years this was me. I didn't think about running as a form of exercise that was for me. I'd rather do an aerobics class at the local leisure centre. Running was something other people did and they seemed, although for the life of me I didn't know why, to enjoy it. 'Leave them to it, that's their thing,' I thought. And left it at that.

2. *OK. Maybe I can try running* (contemplation – getting ready stage)
   Often there is a trigger between the pre-contemplation stage and this stage that makes you consider trying running. What was it – or is it – for you? What triggered you to buy this book? What's making you continue to read these words? As I said in the previous chapter, for me it was that GP appointment and the doctor suggesting I 'try jogging'. And please understand that I didn't take up running immediately: I stayed in the pre-contemplation stage for a while longer – at least until my mental illness made it too damn uncomfortable to stay there.
   
   *During stages 1 and 2 it's important to remember that you can often stay there for a while. You might even go back to pre-contemplation – yes, the yo-yo thing. You may think about what it might be like to try running but consciously and subconsciously feel, or build, barriers that stop you progressing to the next stage.

3. *I'm ready to try running* (preparation – ready stage)
   Many of you reading this book might be between the contemplation and preparation stages. You are on that cusp of wanting to prepare to start running. And that's what this stage of change is about, the *preparation*. Making the decision to start running. That might be buying this book; it might be asking a friend if they fancy learning to run with you; it might be pulling out an old sports bra, a pair of jogging pants and a T-shirt from the cupboard; it might be consciously thinking of a day, week

or month when you might like to start. But, know this: once you make that commitment and start to mentally and physically prepare, then you are moving into the action stage.

4. *Check me out. I'm bloody running!* (action – making change stage)
This is it. This is the stage when you turn to the Miles and Smiles chapter on page 212 and look at 'week one, day one' of that 5K training plan that I have put together for you and you think, 'Right, today is the day.' You get that sports bra on, get those clothes and trainers on and – like I did – you might even clutch that bottle of water in your hand like your life depends on it. You are going to run. *Now, the problem with this action stage – as anybody who has tried not just learning to run, but any form of exercise, will know – is that starting to run feels really bloody hard. You've probably never been shown how to run efficiently, you have no idea about breathing or how to listen to your body, you feel totally out of sorts. This is a critical stage and research shows that it's the time when people can relapse, often quite quickly, maybe even after six to eight weeks (there's a reason my training plan lasts 10 weeks!). This model argues that after six months the behaviour becomes a habit. By then you will have built it into your life through consistency and will have seen mental and physical changes – such as improved mental wellness, increased fitness and improved self-esteem, among a host of other changes – which will spur you on to keep going into the fifth and final stage.

5. *Come, run with me!* (maintenance – keeping up change stage)
This is the stage I want you to get to, and that's what this book is here to help with. Running – in whatever form you move your body – is now a part of your life. No matter what that running looks like. You will see the benefits both small and large that being active and moving your body with joy and purpose can bring to your life and, whether you know it or not, you will be advocating that to other women. They will see you. You will be the representation that they need to see to 'try this running stuff'. Your journey will not only empower you, but it will inspire your family, your friends and people you may never even meet.

I think it's important to say that just because you have graduated on to a higher stage, it does not mean that you can't go back. Hands up who has tried something that they thought had stuck and then life got busy, which led you to take a break or even stop. I know I have.

But going backwards does not mean you have failed. Missing a running practice does not mean you have failed. All runners experience this back and forth. It's part of the runner's life. My training plan is designed for you to start where you are. To progress, to adapt, to progress, to adapt. Because in running, it's in the planned adaptation weeks, and in the rest days, that your body alters and, ultimately, you get stronger, more confident and ready to run once again.

## Safety matters

Women need to feel safe when they go out for a run. It matters.

For me, and the women I work with, 'feeling safe' is up there in the top five reasons why we do not take up running, or we stop running. A report by ASICS called 'Closing the Gender Exercise Gap' cites safety at number three in its list of top-five barriers women face when it comes to exercise. A feeling of 'safety in numbers' is why lots of women tell me they like female-only running groups, and it's also why there has been an increase in online and offline running communities for women only.

You might have anxiety when you're thinking about going out for a run, and question who you should go with, what time you should go, etc. And it's important that you know that you are not alone in feeling this. It IS different for us as women who are new to running. We have to think about safety in a way that males do not. It IS an additional barrier for us.

In chapter 8 I am going to dive into this and share with you all the experience, skills and tips that many women use to stay as safe as they possibly can when running.

# Empowering the runner in YOU

There's been a lot to take on board in this chapter, I know. I am asking you to consider embracing a new identity as a runner, as an athlete (I don't want to use the word 'amateur' – because, girl, there ain't nothing amateur about you!). I am asking you to use words to describe yourself that you might not have considered before. And, it's fair to say that at this stage you may not have even run a step! But my experience shows me that words matter, so these small steps – the first being to use the words 'I am a runner' – matter.

So let's start as we mean to go on. Close your eyes and, with me, breathe in through your nose for a count of five. Now breathe out through your mouth for a count of five. Repeat this process again. Keep your eyes closed and repeat, 'I am a runner.' Now say it louder for those at the back: 'I AM A RUNNER!'

You can also try saying out loud some of these empowering mantras:

- 'I can do hard things.'
- 'I can run strong; I can run free.'
- 'The pain is temporary; the beauty remains.'
- 'Small steps; big strides.'

CHAPTER 3

# Don't sweat the technique

I've been watching professional athletes run for as long as I can remember, from cheering on Tessa Sanderson – the first Black British woman to win an Olympic title in a track and field event – in the 1980s, to shouting at the television with pride as British 400m runner Kelly Holmes won gold in the 2000s.

I've always been intrigued by how top-level runners do what they do. And I don't just mean how fast they run – I know that is a combination of talent, training and time on feet. More than that I've been intrigued by 'how' they run. Because they can look so different.

Each runner has a different running 'form' – a different way they encourage their body to move forwards. They've developed this from years spent practising: they have spent hours and hours working with expert coaches refining their craft.

The techniques they practise aren't secret. They're not locked away in some hidden room where only elite athletes can access them. They are available to you and me too. Understanding them and how you can use them to develop your very own running form is an important part of this journey you are about to go on.

I practise some type of technique every time I run. It helps to ground me, to keep me present and to keep me coming back. Understanding why it's important – and doing it – will help you, too.

# A winning form

If you ever watched marathon running legend Paula Radcliffe in a race you would have seen that, as her body worked harder over each mile, her head-nodding became more pronounced. Now, compare Paula's form with that of the likes of Eliud Kipchoge – one of the greatest male marathon runners of all time – and you'll see a stark contrast: that man just glides like a swan on water.

They have both held world records and won multiple marathons, but their forms could not be more different. Because they are unique – just as you are – they have developed winning forms that work for them, based on a set of principles that you too can learn.

Emma Kirk-Odunubi is a sports scientist, run coach and run analyst. She is also a friend of mine and is known for her informative running content. She says this of technique: 'In my 15-plus years spent analysing the running gait of thousands of people, I can tell you that there is no *right* way to run. Yes, of course, there are attributes and form that help but, ultimately, it's about finding the right way to run *for you*.

'I see people comparing their form to others and beating themselves up because they think they're getting it wrong all the time. I say to them to focus on their mind, their body, their mechanics, what strength work they might need. Understanding this, and applying it, will serve you well.'

I agree wholeheartedly with Emma. One size does not fit all. That said, when learning to run, there are six running technique fundamentals that I have to share with you. By running technique, I mean the way that you hold and move your body when you're running.

It is important that as a new runner you understand and become comfortable practising these during your running sessions. Doing so will improve how energy-efficient you are when you run, and this will make your journey more enjoyable. It will also reduce the risk of injury and you will become a stronger, more resilient runner. Running will become a sustainable habit.

> Around 30–35 per cent of new runners experience injuries in their first year, with improper technique being a major factor.

## It's only natural

We're told that running is natural: it's a natural way for us to move our bodies and something that we, as a species, have done for eons. If we needed food back in the day, long before we could get it delivered to our front doors, we hunted. We ran both solo and in packs because what humans possess is the ability to outrun – over days, weeks or months – all other animals. Over time, this trained our brains to learn that if we keep moving, we get what we want.

But when was the last time you ran to catch your own food? When was the last time you ran for anything that you really wanted? Maybe it was a bus? Maybe it was to stop your toddler from crossing a road?

Once that run was over, what was the thing you had to overcome? I bet it was to recover your breathing. To take a hot moment to catch your breath by standing still and taking in massive gulps of air. Why? Because when you were running you weren't thinking about your breath rate or belly breathing technique. You just wanted to get to where you were going, fast. And that lack of thought is the reason you felt the way you did afterwards. The reason your legs felt like jelly. Why? Because they did not have enough oxygen-rich blood delivered to them. Lactate built up and the only thing that would make them feel normal again was air – and maybe a long sit-down!

The first time I went for a run I felt as if I was losing my breath – that I couldn't inhale enough oxygen to power what I wanted to do. I didn't understand how best to do it. Because, at that time, I had no one to show me. Luckily, you've got me.

# Running technique 101

What are the techniques that will allow you to efficiently 'fall forwards' – which is ultimately what you are doing when running – in a safe and efficient manner?

Here are the key fundamentals when it comes to your practice of running technique that will improve your running form. Don't panic: you will not be expected to do all of these, all at once, on every run. We'll focus on one technique at a time, in order to keep you present in the run and aware of what is happening in your body.

> **'TEETH AND TITS, LADIES, TEETH AND TITS!'**
>
> 'I joined a local running club to learn how to run. The beginners' group was led by a loud, confident woman and I remember, on one of our first sessions, she was explaining the importance of posture when running. In order for us to remember to keep our chest up, she told us to recite the mantra "teeth and tits". As she said tits, she got us to practise running tall, chest proud, ribcage open. And as she said "teeth", we were to "remember to smile". I'll always remember her and, every time I feel tired, her voice comes into my head: "Teeth and tits, ladies, teeth and tits."'

## 1 Posture

Your posture is so important when learning to run. How you hold yourself while moving your body forwards influences everything.

### Why posture matters

- It'll make breathing easier because your chest will be kept open, enabling greater lung capacity and the ability to take on oxygen.
- It will reduce unnecessary side-to-side movements, which in turn will decrease strain on your muscles and joints.

- It will ensure balanced muscle engagement and will prevent other muscles overcompensating, which can lead to injury.
- It will allow you to move forwards efficiently with minimal wasting of energy.
- It'll keep your centre of gravity aligned over your feet, which will help you balance, reducing trips and falls.
- Running, and walking, tall will boost your confidence. A good posture allows us women to signal 'I'm here and I am doing this.' That confident stance – or power pose – will impact how you'll feel physically.

## Ignore posture and . . .

- Your lung capacity will be reduced due to hunching and slouching. This will make it harder to breathe and will limit what you can do.
- You'll get tired and feel discomfort more quickly due to some of your muscles working harder than they need to.

## How to do it

1. Keep your head upright and look forwards. Try not to look down at your feet. I know that you will be worried about tripping and will want to look at the floor, but do practise keeping your head up and your gaze ahead and at the terrain in front of you.
2. Keep your shoulders back and relaxed. If you find yourself hunching your shoulders up towards your ears, intentionally drop them down. I also find shaking out both arms at the sides to release built-up tension can help.
3. Remember 'teeth and tits, ladies!'. Keep your chest open and lifted to encourage better lung capacity.
4. Lean slightly forwards from your ankles, not your hips. This will help your forward momentum.
5. Avoid too much side-to-side movement when swinging your arms (more on this below).
6. Engage your core (more on this below).

> **COACHING TIP**
>
> Pick something ahead of you that is higher up, like a treetop. It'll encourage you to keep your head up, shoulders back and chest open.

## 2 Breathing

The thing that catches so many new runners out is understanding the important partnership between breathing and running. Practising how to regulate your breathing while running takes patience and getting comfortable with it may not come as naturally, or as quickly, as you would like. You will also need to practise tuning into how quickly you are breathing and feeling what part of your body that breath is coming from. For example, are you breathing deeply from your diaphragm/tummy or shallowly from your upper chest/throat?

> **DON'T PANIC!**
>
> 'When I don't listen to my body when I am running, I get into a lot of trouble. I am fairly new to running and, sometimes if I am running with a group, I can get caught up and fall into the trap of trying to go faster than I am able to. My breathing is the first thing to go. It gets shallower and I don't feel I can inhale enough oxygen. Then, as my heart rate gets too high, I get panicky, which can often result in tears. My coach is really on it and reminds me to "go at my pace", to ignore the paces of others. To respond to these cues and to dial it back before they become overwhelming. I am getting better at listening to my body, but it does take practice.'

You want to make sure that your body gets enough oxygen to feed it during each running session, because it will energise your runs and make this process so much more joyful.

## Why breathing matters

- Your working muscles need enough oxygen to do what you are asking of them.
- As a woman, on average you have a smaller lung capacity than a man. You need maximum oxygen to keep fatigue at bay.
- It'll help you to maintain a steady pace for longer and improve the length of time you feel able to run.
- It'll keep your heart rate (HR) stable. Too many HR spikes can cause discomfort and panic. You don't want that.
- You'll feel calmer and more in control, especially during those runs that may demand a little more of you.
- If you practise diaphragmatic (belly) breathing, it'll reduce the likelihood of you getting a side stitch (sharp pain in the abdomen) by allowing for fuller oxygen exchange while reducing the strain on your diaphragm (I'll explain more on p. 32).
- You'll feel more relaxed, which will translate to less tension felt in the neck, shoulders and back. You'll also be a smoother, more efficient runner.
- It'll keep you focused and in tune with your body. You'll be able to spot areas of tension or niggles before they become big problems.

## Ignore breathing and . . .

- Your body will tire more quickly, meaning you'll slow down more.
- You'll be more likely to get a side stitch. These can often be caused by shallow breathing, which is (don't worry!) very common in new runners.
- Your heart rate may elevate too quickly, which can lead to feelings of anxiety or panic and thinking that 'I can't do it.'
- You may overexert yourself, which could lead to injury.
- It'll take you longer to recover after each session, which might affect your consistency.

### How to do it

1. **Belly breathing (diaphragmatic breathing)** – Aim to minimise the amount of shallow (chest) breathing that you are doing when running. Instead, encourage deep breaths that allow maximal oxygen uptake. Belly breathing can help with this. Practise by consciously breathing deeply into your belly rather than shallow breathing into your chest. To check this, place a hand on your abdomen and feel it rise and fall with each breath you take. Take time to practise belly breathing when you are out on a run.
2. **Rhythmic breathing** – This is a way to sync your breathing with your steps. For example:

- Low exertion: 3:2 ratio – inhale for three steps, then exhale for two steps
- Moderate exertion: 2:2 ratio – inhale for two steps, then exhale for two steps
- High exertion: 2:1 ratio – inhale for two steps, then exhale for one step

People often ask me, 'Is it better to breathe through your nose or your mouth?' My answer for beginners is, use both. I find practising breathing through my nose easier during slower, comfortable sessions than I do when I am putting in a bit more effort. When it comes to how to breathe when you are running, everyone has an opinion, but to effectively run and breathe through your nose alone takes a lot of practice and, for this book, it's not something I want you to get tied up worrying about. The main thing is that you are getting enough oxygen in through belly and rhythmic breathing.

Being on this journey of contemplating starting to run will provide the perfect environment for you to build and refine your breathing technique. Why? Because it's easier to practise when you are moving slower and really taking time to feel what's going on in your body. And, as 80 per cent of the running that you do on my programme will be at the low/moderate exertion rate, it's a no-brainer.

## 3 Arm movement

Over the years, I've seen all sorts of interesting arm movements in runners, from arms that flail at the side or swing back and forth faster than the legs are running, to arms that criss-cross the body, creating instability and excessive energy leakage (more on that on page 34). Yes, everyone finds a form of running that works for them, but if those people really understood how their arm movements impacted their running efficiency, endurance and enjoyment, they would likely try to correct it. Personally, arm movement is something that I am hyper-aware of because, when I get tired, it is often the first thing to slide.

### Why arm movement matters

- If your arms are in sync with your legs, they will increase your forward momentum without you having to rely solely on your legs.
- Good arm swing will reduce rotational movements in your upper body, making you a smoother runner.
- You'll feel more stable and in control of how you run.
- You'll be more co-ordinated in your running technique – co-ordination is a key skill for all runners to practise.
- It'll help with overall running posture.

### Ignore arms movement and . . .

- You'll waste valuable energy.
- You're at risk of creating muscle imbalances that can lead to increased fatigue and injury.
- You might find it harder to breathe. Slouched shoulders or clenched fists can lead to tension, which affects lung capacity and thus the amount of time you're able to run.

### How to do it

1. Keep your arms bent, maintaining a 90-degree angle at the elbow.
2. Swing your arms back and forth from the shoulder, ensuring that they are parallel to each other, rather than swinging them

across the front of the body. The opposite arm should move up/forwards at the same time as the opposite leg.
3. Avoid shrugging. Keep your shoulders relaxed and lowered.
4. Try not to clench your hands. Instead, imagine that you are holding a delicate bird's egg, feather or a crisp between your thumbs and forefinger. Think light touch.
5. For easy, comfortable and moderate runs, keep a relaxed arm swing. For runs that require a little more effort, swing your arms a little harder. Think about that co-ordination.

> **ENERGY LEAKAGE**
>
> No, I'm not talking about urinating while on the run! Well, not in this chapter anyway (see chapter 11 for more on the pelvic floor). Leakage, in the context of running technique, refers to the loss of energy or ability to run efficiently. If there is an inefficiency in how the energy that you have available is transferred through the body – for example, you overly rotate your torso when you are running by swinging your arms across the front of your body – then 'leakage' can occur as a result of that. And that leakage can lead to reduced forward motion and increased fatigue. You're basically wasting all of that very useful energy.

## 4 Core engagement

What is your core? If, like so many other runners, you believe that it's just the tummy muscles (abdominals) then you would be wrong (but not alone!). Your core is so much more: it consists of muscles in the back, hips, pelvic floor and diaphragm. And when it comes to running, your 'core engagement' has an impact on all of the above techniques and more.

### Why core engagement matters

- Your core is the central link between your upper and lower body. Engaging it will help to stabilise your spine and pelvis during running.

- If your core is engaged then your upper body won't rotate as much, allowing you to move forwards more easily.
- When you get tired it'll help you maintain balance, especially on uneven ground.
- It'll minimise strain on muscles and joints in the lower back, hips and other areas of the body.
- It'll help you generate more power from every stride and arm swing you make.

## Ignore it and . . .

- You'll find that compensatory movements you make may increase the risk of lower back pain and other niggles.
- You will experience excessive energy leakage.
- You might feel unstable.
- You'll experience more of a tendency to slouch, which will affect posture, lung capacity and make the run feel harder.

## How to do it

1. When you're running, think about tightening your lower abdominals by focusing on the area just below your belly button. Gently draw in your belly button towards your lower spine. I don't want you to suck it in completely, because that will restrict your breathing: just gently pull.
2. Another tip is to imagine that you are gently tightening a corset around your core. With each pull of those corset strings, your core is tightening.
3. Imagine if someone was readying themselves to prod you in the tummy. You'd brace a little, wouldn't you? Tighten up. That feeling is the start of core engagement.
4. The key thing when it comes to core engagement is to remember to do it while running. It's something that, when coaching female runners, I'll enthusiastically remind them about every five minutes: 'Cor blimey, ladies! Remember your core!' Find a prompt that works for you or use mine.

Core strengthening exercises that you can do to support your running can be found in chapter 11.

## 5 Stride length and cadence

Put simply, stride length is the amount of ground that you will cover with each step that you take. Cadence refers to how many steps you take, normally per minute, when running. And they both work in partnership: faster cadence, shorter stride = less likelihood of injury.

Emma says of this: 'Cadence is the biggest indicator for people getting injured. There is no one cadence that you should hit but, if your cadence is not within a range of, say, 160–180 steps per minute (SPM) there is a stronger likelihood of injury. For brand-new runners I'd advise trying to run with lighter feet. Why? Because when you try to do this, your feet will naturally turn over faster. It's unlikely that I'll see people who are running "light" with a low cadence. Imagine you are running on hot coals.'

### Why stride length and cadence matter

- If you focus on increasing your cadence – meaning taking shorter strides and more of them each minute – you may find you can run a little more quickly.
- If you aim for a cadence between 160 and 180 SPM it'll mean more efficient running. A key point to remember is that, as a new runner, your cadence will more likely be towards the 160 number because you'll be running slower.
- Shorter steps with higher cadence will reduce feelings of fatigue.

### Ignore it and . . .

- You might try to cover too much ground with each stride, which will waste energy.
- You might be unknowingly applying too much force through your leg on each stride, which can lead to injury.

## How to do it

1. When you are running, try to ensure that your foot – on each step you take – lands underneath your body, rather than ahead of it.
2. Stay tall. Running with good posture, and staying relaxed, will help you achieve the right stride length for you.
3. If you want to measure your cadence, count the number of steps you take in 15 seconds and multiply that by four. That will tell you what your current cadence is. If you want to aim to get within the 160–180 SPM range, aim to increase by 5–10 per cent slowly, to avoid strain.

## 6 Foot strike

When you run, the way that your foot makes contact with the ground is called 'foot strike'. When it comes to running, there are three different ways that runners tend to land:

1. **Heel** – Your heel will make the first contact with the ground (often seen in new runners).
2. **Midfoot** – The middle of your foot lands, almost flat, on the ground.
3. **Forefoot** – The ball of the foot makes first contact with the ground (often seen in sprinters).

There is a common misconception that heel striking – something many new runners tend to do – is wrong. It's not.

Emma says: 'I have looked at thousands of runners over the years using a high-tech piece of equipment called MotionMetrix. This helps me to analyse people when they are running – looking at their joint angles, foot strike, basically everything I'd need to know as a run analyst.

'When you are fatigued as a runner, even an elite runner, you will tend to heel strike. Anatomically some people – due to the lengths and angles of their bones – will always naturally heel strike. For me, the focus is on helping runners to practise landing their feet just underneath their body, rather than saying, "Don't heel strike."

'If you are running in an efficient motion and still achieving that falling-forward action then why is how your foot strikes wrong? Everyone runs differently. It's to do with your own anatomical make-up. Your female bone structure will determine how your body moves. Find a way to run that works for you and, if it doesn't or results in niggles, seek advice.'

As new runners, a higher proportion of you will tend to heel strike when you start. Why? Well, a) you will be running slower – and slower running can encourage heel striking; and b) you are new to practising your running – no one has shown you any different.

So, if during the process of learning to run, you experience niggles or injury, I want you to think to yourself, 'Could this be due to how I am landing and, if so, how can I resolve it?'

## Why foot strike matters

- Developing a natural, efficient and comfortable foot strike *for you* will equate to less discomfort and fatigue, resulting in more enjoyable running.
- Understanding your foot strike and how that impacts on your body, both positively and negatively, will feed into the decisions you make during each session on what elements of technique to practise.

## Ignore it and . . .

- You may experience niggles or injury associated with excessive impact force through your lower body. This is associated with heavy heel strike, for example.
- You may experience calf and Achilles tendon strain, which can be associated with a higher tendency to forefoot run.
- You might overly tense your feet and ankles, which can lead to discomfort and injury.

## How to do it

1. With every step you take, make it your aim to land softly and quietly. Tune into the foot. Where does it feel like you are landing with each step? Heel, midfoot or forefoot?
2. Try to ensure your foot lands underneath your body, *not ahead of it*. You many need to shorten your stride to achieve this.
3. Running with a slight forward lean, as if you are almost falling forwards – from the ankles not the hips – will encourage a more natural foot strike for you.

Studies show that one of the reasons runners tend to get injured is because they didn't have anyone to help them to understand technique or to answer questions that they have. I don't want that to be you.

Practising some of these techniques during this amazing running journey you are about to go on will help to build a form of running that works for you.

You were made for this!

CHAPTER 4

# Gearing up to run

This chapter isn't about me telling you that you need to go out and spend hundreds of pounds on the latest carbon-plated running shoes or technical compression gear. You don't! It's also not about baffling you with pseudoscience that, in all reality, is marketing spiel designed to scare you and build a culture of one-up-woman ship among us amateur runners.

This chapter is me being that friend to you, the one I didn't have when I went out for my first run in 2009. I want to offer you advice as a coach and a runner on what has worked well for me, and others, and what gear it might be worth trying. I'm going to go back in time and remember all the questions that I had – and the questions that I regularly answer from women who are starting to run.

So, when it comes to gear, I am going to list all that you as a new runner need, from most important to least important.

> The estimated value of the global running gear market by 2033 is $66.9 billion.

## 1 Shoes

### It takes more than a pair of shoes!
When I talk to people about barriers to access for women who want to learn to run, I am often met with the response, 'What's the problem? All it takes is a pair of shoes!' That is just not true.

There *are* visible and invisible barriers that exist for you, much more so than for men. And, yes, although trainers are a very important piece of kit, having the confidence to learn to run is about so much more than owning a pair.

But since they are a very important piece of kit, as part of your running journey, there is going to come a point when you will want to think about the shoes you are wearing. Because wearing trainers that work 'with' not 'against' the make-up of your foot, that support how you land and take off, can make a massive difference to your enjoyment of running.

Running in shoes that do not give your feet the support they need can lead to niggles, which can lead to injury, which can lead to you having to stop running in order to rehabilitate yourself.

## Do you already have trainers?

If you do, what I want you to do is go and grab that pair of trainers that you have used for *any* form of exercise (this includes walking the dog, taking the kids to school and walking to the local cafe). Hold them up in front of you and have a good look at them. What do you see when you look at the underside of the trainer? How worn down are the lugs (the bumpy bits that are on the underside of the trainer and have been designed to give you a bit of grip)? Can you see more wear on a particular part of the lugs on the right-hand or left-hand side, toe or heel? Now turn them over and look at the top of the trainer. Are there any signs of wear and tear there? For example, on the area where the outside of your foot would be, near your little toe? Or where your big toe would be? Can you notice any holes or worn fabric?

Why am I asking you to do this? Well, because it will make the terminology a little bit clearer. And – should you decide to take my advice and venture into a sports shop and ask for some help – you may be asked similar questions.

> ### WHAT DOES 'RUNNING GAIT' MEAN?
>
> It means pronation: the natural movement of your foot as it interacts with the ground when you land. There are three different types of pronation: **neutral**, **overpronation** or **underpronation** (also called **supination**).

Depending on the amount of time you have owned, and used, your trainers, looking at them closely may give you an indication as to what your gait is.

## Neutral
The wear on the underside of your shoe is equally distributed. This means:

- Your foot rolls inwards about 15 per cent.
- Impact forces are optimally distributed when landing.
- A neutral shoe would provide you with adequate support.

## Overpronation
The wear on the underside of your shoe is more visible on the inner edges (big toe side) of your trainer. This means:

- Your foot rolls inwards more than 15 per cent.
- This is common in people with flatter feet.
- Stability shoes can help to evenly distribute impact.

## Underpronation (supination)
The wear on the underside of your trainer is more visible on the outer edge (little toe side) of your trainer. This means:

- Your foot rolls inwards less than 15 per cent.
- This is common in people with high arches.
- Extra cushioning can help absorb impact.

## Leave it to the experts!

You do not need to go out and buy a pair of brand-new trainers to start running – hell no. And many women don't. They start running in what they have, to see how they get on. I often find that, after a couple of weeks, they get a feel as to whether this form of exercise is something they can enjoy and – if so – that is often the time when they start asking me about upgrading trainers, or they start to feel niggles emanating from trainers that need to be upgraded. That is the time to seek expert help.

If you feel that you want some expert support, look up a local sports shop – preferably one that sells a variety of running trainers. Give them a call and ask them whether they offer gait analysis. This basically means they will have a running machine that is set up with a camera that can film how your feet hit the treadmill. You will have to get on the machine and jog for a couple of minutes for them to get the data they need but, once they have it, they will be able to tell you what your gait is and, better than that, they will be able to pull out a load of trainers that have been designed specifically for your gait.

If the idea of going into a shop and running in front of strangers, on a machine that feels foreign, while being filmed at the same time, puts the fear of God into you, then go online and search 'run analyst'. There are a host of amazing female experts – my friend Emma Kirk-Odunubi being one of them – who offer consultations for runners looking to find the right shoe for them.

Emma again: 'I offer an online gait analysis service for those people who don't want, or don't have the time, to go instore. I'll ask people to send me a video of them running down a street (filmed by someone else), which I can analyse and feed back on. Also, by seeing how their feet move via live videoconferencing, I can then suggest the best shape and function of running shoe that might work for them.'

Many sports shops offer this analysis free of charge in the hope that you will buy a pair of trainers from them.

## Nice toes, naughty toes

Everyone's feet are different – and how we use them changes due to our bespoke genetic and life history. I have very wide feet, which means that, for a long time, I struggled to find a pair of trainers that allowed enough room for my forefoot to expand on impact with the ground without causing my little toes to rub on the outer edge of my trainer, causing the dreaded blister. Back in the day it seemed that many sports brands only produced wide-fitting trainers in shoes that were marketed to men. But in the past few years many brands have become wiser to the needs of the female runner, although *much* more still needs to be done. I always look for a trainer with an ample toe box – that's the part of the trainer that forms the area where your forefoot and toes are. I know some of the same struggles apply to female runners with narrow feet – their trainers are often too roomy in the toe box, causing their foot to slide about inside the trainer, again causing blisters.

My advice to you is try, try and try again. And that's why, for your first pair of trainers, I would suggest visiting an actual running-shoe shop. Often the good ones, the ones that really understand runners, will let you run up and down the street outside the shop to test out how the trainers feel.

## You're doing SWELL, honey

When picking a pair of trainers, I would always advise going half a shoe size, or even a whole shoe size, bigger than your normal size. Why? Because when you run, your feet will expand and swell, so you need more room in your trainers. A good rule of thumb is to have half to a full thumb's width of space between your toes and the end of your trainer.

It's also important to remember that, while you may need more room in the toe box for swelling, your heels should fit more snugly than they do in normal shoes. The last thing you want is for your heel to be moving from side to side, which can potentially cause injury and, I'll say it again, more blisters.

As we get older, our feet can become flatter and wider due to weight gain (blasted menopause!), injuries and pregnancy. As you get into your running I'd really recommend getting your feet remeasured when you buy your trainers and then again *at least once a year*. Feet measuring isn't just for the kids at the start of the school year.

> **THE SHOES OFF HIS OWN FEET!**
>
> 'I was doing a longer-distance event and my feet really swelled up to the point that every step I took felt like a hot poker was prodding the side of my foot. I knew I needed to change my trainers but didn't have larger ones with me. My husband was waiting to cheer me on. When he saw my pain and my need for a bigger size of trainer, he took off his trainers and gave them to me. Of course, this gave my toes more room and reduced the pain. I may have only been able to shuffle and walk to the finish line but – at that point, I couldn't have loved him more!'

## Terrain

Another question that you will get asked when selecting a pair of trainers is, 'What type of terrain will you be running on?' Why does it matter? Because – yes, you've guessed it – trainers are made for different types of surface.

Now, for the majority of you reading this book as beginners, or as returners to running, I am going to assume that you will be running on either road (tarmac or other artificial surfaces) or trail (off-road surfaces like grass, flat hard-packed dirt surfaces or woodland). The great news for you is that there are trainers designed for them all. And, to put it simply, here's the difference:

**Road shoes** – These are designed to be used to run on smooth, hard and even surfaces like pavements and roads. They normally have smoother, flatter outsoles for traction and softer midsoles for more cushioning. Many road shoes available these days incorporate wider toe boxes for additional comfort.

**Trail shoes** – These are designed to be used on softer, more uneven and changeable ground. They often have larger (up to 5mm/⅕in) and softer lugs on the outsole for better grip on uneven terrain. Their midsole is often stiffer, which will provide you with more stability on trails. They'll often feel like a tighter fit to your foot, which will give you more control over trail terrain. Some brands of trail shoe also feature toe guards and hidden plates that will protect your feet against rocks and roots.

**Hybrid shoes** – These are a type of running shoe that give you the best of both worlds. They have been designed to provide versatility for runners who want to easily transition between road running and trail running.

If you are buying a pair of trainers, then you will see that there are male and female versions. 'Does it matter?' I hear you ask. Well, when it comes to many of the ranges available, the answer is 'Not really', because historically trainer design has been based on male feet. The female versions are basically shrunken-down versions of these and come in, for some of us, annoying pastel colours. The shoe you pick to run in will depend on your foot size, shape and comfort preferences, not whether they are designated as being for men or women.

From a biomechanical point of view, women's feet tend to be narrower in the heel and midfoot but wider in the forefoot and toe area compared to men's feet of the same size. We also generally have smaller feet compared to men.

If you are trying on trainers, try as many as you can and find what works for you.

### SUSTAINABLE RUNNING

The idea that running shoes should be replaced after 500–800km (300–500 miles) is a myth created by corporations looking to profit from misinformation. You should use other metrics to assess whether your trainers are suitable. Some signs that your running shoes need to be replaced include:
- You are experiencing pain in the knees, hips and shins.
- Your trainers feel heavy, flat or don't have enough bounce.
- The cushioning inside has deteriorated.
- They are full of holes.
- The lugs are badly worn in some areas, which will affect grip.

# 2 Sports bras

## Over-the-shoulder boulder-holder

Knowing what to wear and how to support and care for your breasts can be a barrier to exercise for some women. Your sports bra should be your best friend but, depending on how well you choose it, it can hinder rather than help.

So that's why I'm listing it second on the list of essential gear for beginner runners. Because your sports bra matters. It's a must-have.

For context, right now I am a DD cup. I have been a B cup and a C cup in my running lifetime. On my first run, my girls (and yes, I do refer to my boobs as 'my girls'), were held down the best they could be in a maternity bra. It's all I had and was the most supportive bra that I could wear at the time.

I had too much to think about in getting ready for that first jog and, in all reality, my boobs bouncing up and down was the least of my worries. But keeping your breasts supported is really important. I have learned a lot – and tried out a lot of bras – in the years since.

We are all unique; our breasts are different and that's OK. They come in different sizes and different shapes. Hey, on certain days my boobs have their own personalities! But not having a supportive bra can make or break your running practice. So, why do you need one and what do you need to consider when buying one?

> **BREAST FACT 1**
>
> The average breast size in the UK is 36DD, which equates to roughly 750g (1lb 11oz) per breast. This means that many of us are carrying around an extra 1.5kg (3lb 5oz) of weight!

Cooper ligaments are the fibrous connections between the inner side of the breast skin and the pectoral muscles. These ligaments work in conjunction with the fatty tissues and more fibrous tissues of the breast, and they are largely responsible for maintaining shape and configuration. As we know, when we move – and certainly when we move quickly – our breasts can move independently of whatever the rest of our bodies are doing.

So, bearing all of this in mind, we want to give our breasts all of the support they need when we are planning on starting to move our bodies in a way that it may not be used to, at a pace which – for many of you – will be new.

I hate that use of the word 'weak' because, actually, our breasts give us so much. And, for the mothers out there who have breastfed their babies even if only for a few minutes, they are life-giving pieces of female kit.

We need a good sports bra to uplift them, to give them support and limit their movement when we are running.

> ### BREAST FACT 2
>
> If the breast moves 60 per cent or more from its natural position during exercise, then immediate, short- and long-term effects can occur.
> - Immediate – You may feel discomfort and pain.
> - Short-term (weeks to months) – You may experience skin irritation and soft tissue strain.
> - Long-term (months to years) – You may experience permanent skin stretching and sagging, musculoskeletal pain and postural issues.

Not wearing a bra that is designed to give your breasts the support they need can lead to breast pain (mastalgia) and breast sag (breast ptosis). I don't want the process of learning to run to cause you pain or unnecessary drop when it doesn't have to. I am here to make that running journey joyful and part of that joy is about making running feel easier on you. Not wearing a sports bra can have an effect on your performance (and every time you go out you are, in a sense, performing).

I don't want you to have to work harder on a run because you don't have the right bra on. If your breasts are left to their own devices on a run without proper support, then your body will increase its use of your upper body muscles. That will mean you have to use more energy, which will make running feel harder.

Consequences of not wearing a sports bra include:

- Breast pain
- Breast sag
- Negatively affected performance
- Changes to breathing pattern (due to more pressure on the ribcage)
- Changes to running gait

## How do I pick the right sports bra?

Whether you are a large-, medium- or small-breasted woman, having adequate breast support is important and should be taken seriously.

There are different categories of sports bra. That's the first thing about choosing one that I want you to understand. They are often classified as being suitable for low-, medium- and high-impact activities. I would advise that you look for a high-impact running bra.

## Different types of sports bras for running

**Encapsulation** – My favourite kind. These bras have two cups, like a normal bra. They also tend to come in the same sizes as regular bras – which is a bonus.

**Compression** – These look more like a crop top. They work by pressing your breasts against your chest and are usually pulled on over your head. They tend to be a good option for smaller-breasted women. Top tip: if you are opting for a compression bra, make sure the centrepiece lies flat against your breastbone, to avoid chafing. Compression bras tend to come in small, medium, large and extra large (which can be uncomfortable to wear/not give the right support if you have small breasts but a large chest band size).

**Combination** – These combine the qualities of the other two types in order to provide the highest level of support. These are good bras for larger-breasted women.

Whether you are going into a shop to try on a sports bra or you have ordered one online to try at home, I want you to replicate the movement pattern that you will be doing. That means jogging – so jog on the spot and see how it feels, lift your arms up, circle them around, rotate your torso from side to side, touch your toes. How does the sports bra feel on you?

There are so many different types of running bras on the market and it has taken me years to find ones that work better for me. Personally, I like a racer-back sports bra that has separate cups for my breasts to sit in. I also like bras with a soft underside on the chest band as, when running, I suffer badly with chafing – *see* p. 60 for more on ways to counter that affliction.

However, there is no single correct method for bra fitting. The most common method we as women have been using to check chest and cup sizes (when you measure over the bust for the cup size and around the chest for the band size) varies greatly from country to country, brand to brand and woman to woman. So, when you are trying on a sports bra, remember these points:

**Band** – Check that it is firm (with about 2.5–5cm/1–2in of give) and level around your chest. It should move with you, not independent of you. If it is adjustable, which many of them are, start on the loosest setting.

**Shoulder strap** – Again, aim for 2.5–5cm/1–2in of give and ensure the straps don't fall off your shoulders or dig into you. Racer-back (cross-strap) bras are great for extra support, too.

**Cup** – Always check that your breasts fill the whole cup – if it is a bra that has separate cups – and there is no bulging or wrinkling of the material.

**Underwire** – If the bra has underwires, then ensure that the wire is not sitting on the breast tissue itself at the front or under the arm.

**Supportive** – Remember to try all the movement patterns I have listed above, to check it is supportive enough.

**Comfortable** – It should be comfortable. We don't need an uncomfortable bra diminishing our running joy.

> ### SPORTS BRA CONTORTION!
>
> 'When choosing a sports bra, a key part to decision-making is asking, "How easily can I get it on and off?" I've lost track of how many times I've been stuck trying to get a sports bra off over my head, especially those higher-support ones. That's why I love sports bras with zips at the front – game-changer!'

Most but not all – and again it depends on the brand and the amount of money that you are paying – running bras are made of technical fabrics that wick (move away) sweat and moisture from the skin, thus keeping you cool and dry and reducing the chances of chafing.

## Bras for post mastectomy and reconstruction surgery

In 2022, an estimated 2.3 million women were diagnosed with breast cancer worldwide. You may be a woman who has been diagnosed, or is living with a diagnosis of, breast cancer. Maybe you have had to decide, with medical support, to have part or the entirety of your breast tissue removed.

My friend Vicky was diagnosed with Stage 1 breast cancer in one breast in 2002 and, in 2006, was diagnosed with Stage 1 breast cancer in the opposite breast. She is now living with Stage 4 cancer, which was diagnosed in 2021. I met Vicky through running.

> **TRY BEFORE YOU BUY**
>
> Vicky: 'When you are living with cancer, you feel as though your body has been completely taken over due to all of the treatment you have. The chemotherapy, the radiotherapy, etc. If, like me, you are someone who was used to being active, I think that not being able to do those things that were good for you mentally and physically – like running – can really mess with your mind. Running post-diagnosis allowed me the opportunity to get some control over my body again, which is so important. I always struggled to find decent sports bras that were comfortable and reflected the shape I wanted. For me, that was to have a breast shape and it was something that I did struggle with – finding a bra that gave me that silhouette. Many of the bras that I tried were heavy, didn't feature underwires (due to no breast to support), felt clunky and not comfortable at all. I did find one from an online store that was great, but they stopped making it. I've still got it to this day. I feel the sports bra market for women who have undergone surgery for breast cancer does need to continue to improve. A lot of the bras are quite expensive, apart from the ones you can pick up in department stores. Therefore, unless you are prepared to spend quite a lot of money, your choice is limited. My advice would be to visit a decent department store, or order from a shop that sells sports bras for women who have had single or double mastectomies – and definitely try before you buy.'

# 3 Clothing

So what do you need to run in? The answer is, what works for you. On my first run I didn't have a single 'running' item in my cupboard so I went out and shuffle/walked in what I had. Did the clothing I was wearing stop me getting out of the door? No. Did it stop me completing that first mile? No. Could it have been more comfortable in the sense of allowing my skin to breathe better, in supporting my boobs, in allowing me to layer up and down as my body temperature dictated? Yes.

You do not need to go out and spend hundreds of pounds on running clothing. If you do not have anything in your cupboard that meets the advice below, then why not try to source some kit from one of the many online second-hand clothing sites there are? Items are normally sold at a quarter of the price and many items are hardly worn (believe me, I use these sites to buy and sell).

## Technical running clothing

The term 'technical' refers to clothing that is designed specifically for running. These items are normally made from fabrics that enhance comfort, breathability and moisture management. They are different to casual workout gear because they can help to regulate your body temperature, wick sweat away from your body and reduce chafing (rubbing/sore bits). Please remember, they are not must-haves (as they can be pricey); this is just so that you know what is out there. Terms you might come across include:

- **Material** – Synthetic fabrics like polyester, nylon or spandex pull (wick) sweat away from your skin, keeping you drier. The fabric dries quickly, which helps prevent chafing.
- **Ventilation** – Items can feature mesh panels or lightweight material that allows airflow, preventing overheating.
- **Flexibility** – This refers to material that allows for a form-fitting design that moves with your body.
- **Compression** – Compression leggings, shorts or socks can help to improve circulation and reduce muscle fatigue.
- **Reflection** – Items with reflective qualities feature built-in reflective panels to ensure visibility in low-light conditions.
- **UV and weather resistance** – These refer to fabrics with UV protection for sunny conditions or showerproof, waterproof or windproof fabric for harsher conditions.

There will always be discussions around what is deemed as 'the best' workout attire, and social media feeds this. There's currently debate about baggy v tight clothing – Gen Z report as preferring baggy clothing, whereas Millennials prefer tight clothing. A 'Year In Sport' report by Strava in 2025 also stated that there are also generational divides on sock length, with Gen Z favouring a crew sock and Gen X voting for a no-show sock.

My advice is: find what works for you! Some days you might like a tight top, on others you'll opt for baggy. Your clothing choice will depend on how you feel mentally, physically and hormonally. I know that if I am feeling bloated, I'll opt for a baggy T-shirt and loose-fitting shorts. Wear what makes you feel good and is made to work with your body from a technical point of view, rather than against it. By adhering to that, you can't go wrong.

When it comes to clothing, I would recommend the following:

- **Leggings (full-or three-quarter-length)** – In colder weather you might want to choose some full-length or three-quarter-length leggings. I like a legging with a high waist to 'hold me in'. Leggings that are designed as 'activewear' often incorporate side pockets or zipped pockets at the back of the waistband for storing small items like keys, money and a phone. So, look at the details and think about what you want.
- **Shorts or skorts** – Do you want to know how many times I have heard women say, 'You'll never catch me in a pair of shorts' and then, a few months later, I see them running around owning it. And I LOVE IT! Life is too damn short to not wear shorts. You're going to get hot so why not let your skin cool quickly by being exposed to the air? I love a pair of figure-hugging running shorts that look like cycling shorts. I own loads of pairs. I like them because a) they have a high waist, b) they come in different leg lengths (one pair ends mid-thigh and another above the knee), and c) wearing them means that I don't suffer chafe when my thighs rub together. You can get loose shorts, tight shorts, short shorts and long shorts. You can also buy a skort, which is a short with a skirt (almost like a tennis skirt) over the top.
- **Top** – You want a T-shirt or a vest that is lightweight and moisture-wicking to keep you dry and comfortable. How tight or loose these are is your call. I don't like really tight tops as I feel constricted,

so I always opt for a size larger than I am. If running in colder weather you might want to opt for a long-sleeved top. Go for one that you can roll the arms up on if you get too hot. I like to layer and use arm sleeves (see page 56) to quickly get warmer/cooler.

- **Jacket** – For rainy, windy or colder days you might want to look at getting a water-resistant or windproof running jacket. They aren't a must, since in the programme you are following with me, you won't be out for hours and hours. But these jackets can be a good investment and mean that there is one less excuse for you to use to *not* go out on a run. 'Oh, I don't have a jacket. I can't go out in this.'
- **Socks** – I hate getting blisters and they can be avoided by choosing the right pair of socks. Blisters often happen when a point on the foot is coming into constant contact with a part of your trainer and causing a 'hot spot'. If not addressed, the hot spot forms a blister and can be incredibly painful to run on. There are hundreds of socks on the market that pride themselves on blister prevention but my advice to you is to experiment. Blister socks don't work for me as my feet get really hot when I run and often the blister socks I have tried are thicker, which exacerbates the problem. I like to run in a thin sock that allows my foot to breathe and provides additional thickness just in the areas where I am likely to feel hot spots. You want to look for running socks that are made from synthetic materials or Merino wool and try to avoid cotton socks, as they retain moisture and can cause issues.

## Nice-to-haves

Below are a couple of items that aren't essential, but are definitely nice to have:

- **Headband or buff** – I LOVE me a buff. My buff and high ponytail have become a bit of a trademark, but I only wear the buff – a large piece of material that can be worn in a multitude of ways – because of the versatility it gives me. It helps to soak up sweat from my forehead, keeps my ears warm and can act like a hat.

I think some form of item for your head to keep sweat out of your eyes, or to keep you a bit warmer, is a good idea.
- **Gloves** – For colder days you might want to invest in a pair of gloves. Again, they don't have to be expensive, and they can also double up as a reflective item if you are running in darker conditions. Many women I know suffer with Raynaud's syndrome – a condition where small blood vessels in your fingers and toes overreact to cold or stress, causing them to temporarily narrow. This leads to reduced blood flow, resulting in colour changes (fingers can often turn white), numbness, tingling and pain or throbbing as circulation returns.
- **Arm sleeves** – These are individual sleeves (kind of like a tight leg warmer, but for your arms) that you can wear. They cover your arms from your wrists to your upper bicep. If it's colder when you start running, you can put them on and, as you get hotter, pull them off easily and store them away. I love mine.
- **Sunglasses** – To protect your eyes from glare and UV rays but also to keep those pesky bugs from flying into your eyes as much as the sun itself!

## Layering

When it comes to clothing for a run, for me it's all about layering. I don't want to overheat or be too cold, so I layer up or down to avoid this. For me that might look like wearing a technical T-shirt, some arm sleeves, a jacket and shorts at the start of a run (depending on the weather) and then – as I get warmer – off comes the jacket, the arm sleeves, etc. I'll store them in my running belt or backpack (or tie them around my waist) and continue on my run.

## Second-hand items

A confession – I have too much running gear. I have bought and been gifted so many items over the years that my closet is overflowing. And do you know what I have found? There are a few favourite pieces that I always come back to. The ones that really work for me. So, I have started selling those I don't need. The second-hand clothing market is booming, as it should be – we have a planet to save. I am an absolute advocate of buying second-hand clothing items (buy some of mine!), especially if you are new to running. Who knows whether you will like running long term (although it's my job to persuade you to), so start by investing small and build your clothing collection from there.

That said, when it comes to trainers, some words of caution about buying second-hand. Your feet are *yours*. When someone wears a pair of trainers, over time, they will mould to the contours of their feet. If you've ever had a pair of shoes that feel like a pair of slippers then you will know what I mean! If you are buying a pair of trainers second-hand, you need to understand how well-worn they are as, if they have moulded to someone else's foot shape, they may be troublesome for you. Also, due to how that person lands when they run, they may have worn down in areas of the outer sole that impact negatively on you. I therefore advise you save money by buying second-hand clothing rather than second-hand trainers.

Emma agrees: 'It's important to know how many miles the previous owner has done. If someone has only put 200 miles into a pair of shoes, then they may work OK for you. All I can say it try them and see. You can tell a lot by looking at the shoe as to what state of use it is in. Does it look worn? What's the tread like? If you are buying a £20 pair of trainers second-hand because you don't know if you want to commit to running then, again, see how you get on but – if you do find you want to continue – I'd advise you to invest in a new pair.'

# 4 Storage

### But what about my stuff?!

The thing I'm asked about the most when I am coaching women during their weekly run practice sessions is where they can store their stuff . . . their bits and bobs.

They'll say to me – often in chorus – 'Sab, I don't have a pocket to store my keys/phone/bank card. Can you look after it for me please?' And, being the supportive running coach I am, I will often let them put these things in my bum bag (fanny pack for my American readers) or my backpack. I will literally take on their load.

But I'm not going to be able to do that for you, so the best I can do is give you some advice on how to select the best bum bags/fanny packs. Because having somewhere secure to store *at least* your phone as you run is really important. Later in this book I am going to talk about a really important topic for us women when we go out running – safety – and one of the key things I will be saying to you is that you *must* carry a fully charged phone.

I don't really want you to be carrying that phone in your hand, gripping on to it for dear life, not only because it will impact on your running form but also because it's something else for you to think about when, in fact, I want you to be thinking about your body and how it is moving. You'll also likely make it all sweaty, which isn't ideal, and could drop it.

> **DON'T USE YOUR BRA AS A POCKET**
>
> 'I remember, I was running my first 5K Parkrun and didn't have anywhere to put my car keys. "Aha," I thought, "I'll shove them down my cleavage right in between my boobs!" I didn't think much about it until I got home and got in the shower. The keys had dug into my boobs, causing marks and, when water hit the damaged skin, I screamed! I made sure to never store them there again and invested in a running belt.'

## Bum bags

I use a bum bag for 5K and 10K runs. I like to keep what I am wearing to hold my stuff within easy reach and as light as possible. If I know that I am not going to need to take water or a substantial amount of food, I can get away with something that I can wear on my waist with minimal storage space.

These packs tend to come in a host of different sizes and have different features. Some are small and compact, designed more as waist belts – see below – with compartments for valuables like phones and car keys. Other packs are purpose-designed to carry a small water bottle. All can be adjusted to fit around your waist in a comfortable manner and can be tightened to stop jiggling while on the move. I have run for years with an Inov-8 bum bag, but there are other variations, too.

## Running belts

There are running belts that have been designed with ease of use in mind for those new to running. They come in different widths and are worn on the waist and designed to minimise the risk of bounce and chafing (there it is again!) that can often come with high-impact exercise.

Most running belts have several compartments for storage and are available in different materials and colours. When selecting a belt, look for a compartment that is big enough to carry your phone and other bits. You will wear your running belt either over or under your T-shirt. Either way, look for a belt made with a fabric that is breathable and doesn't retain moisture, which causes skin irritation.

## Backpacks

If I am running over 10K then I tend to use a running backpack, as it is likely I will want to carry some water, maybe a snack and – if the weather is looking unreliable – I might want to store a light waterproof jacket in my bag. I like a backpack because they often have a multitude of pockets and compartments that have been located in specific areas for ease of access while you are 'on the run'. Also, some women I know – even when training for 5K – like the security of running with a backpack: they say they feel naked without one. Comments such as 'It just feels like another layer of armour' are common.

When choosing a backpack, think about the following:

- It should be light.
- It should feature at least one pocket on the left- or right-hand side of the chest (usually over the breast) that can fit a 500ml (17fl oz) water bottle or soft flask (they sometimes come with these).

- It should be made of fabric that allows sweat to wick from your body.
- It should not hang low on your back or rest on your lower spine.
- It should feature adjustable straps that can be tightened/loosened to ensure a snug fit, eliminating bounce.

### Arm holder

Personally, I am not a fan of an arm holder for the storage of phones or keys. But if you want to wear one, be my guest. You'll still be a runner. I think I was put off them because, in my early running days, I tried a few and they would never stay on my bicep tightly enough, resulting in them slipping down and me having to constantly retighten the band. I am also not a fan of adding additional weight to a particular side of the body when running as I think that, ultimately, it could lead to unnecessary niggles due to other muscle groups overcompensating for the imbalance. That's why I prefer using the above products.

## 5 Chafe management

### For chafe's sake!

For any runner, there are few things worse than chafing. Chafing happens when your skin consistently rubs on another section of your skin (like your inner thighs) or a piece of fabric. This rubbing causes the area to become raw, sore and – in extreme cases – can cause bleeding. (You may have seen male runners with blood seeping through the nipple area of their vests while running. This is due to chafe.)

For me, as a curvy woman, my chafing tends to happen between my thighs (especially if I am wearing shorts that enable my inner thighs to rub together or longer shorts that ride up, exposing the skin). I also get it under my arms (where my bingo wings rub against the sides of my body) and where the chest band of my sports bra sits. And, if I get really sweaty, I get it on my waist (due to the waistband of my shorts getting too sweaty and irritating my skin).

Let me tell you, you'll know if you have been chafed because when you get into the bath or shower after your run, you will feel an intense burning sensation. I have been known to scream upon water contact. I have tried all kinds of creams and lotions over the years but, of late, I have been using one called Bum Butter! (Stop laughing.) Old-school favourites such as Vaseline can also work and, for post-chafe care, Sudocrem or a nappy rash cream helps healing.

I would advise, strongly, that if you are worried about chafing, you should apply Vaseline, Bum Butter or any other anti-chafing lotion before you go out on your run. And if you are unsure what areas to focus on, use my guidance above as a starter for ten. Tip: you can never have too much on! Another thing that works for me is taping chafe-prone areas with KT tape.

## Taping

Kinesiology tape (often referred to as KT tape) is a stretchy tape that is used by runners around the globe to alleviate symptoms of injury. If you have ever watched a race then you may have seen runners with different-coloured tape in mysterious configurations on their body – around their knees, ankles, etc. – that's KT tape. I've been using this for a few years as a fail-safe option to alleviate chafe.

Before I go out on a run I will normally cut KT tape and apply it to my skin directly under the area where the chest strap of my bra will sit and, if I know I will be getting pretty sweaty, I will apply it around the circumference of my hips, too. Often, I'll need to rope in my husband, or the kids, to help me apply it but it really is worth it if you are susceptible to chafing like I am. It might seem like a pretty extreme measure but I have scars on my body where I have chafed badly, so now I've found something that works, I'm going to keep using it – and tell others about it. There are different brands of KT tape but they all do the same thing. A quick search online will deliver you a host of results.

As a word of caution, though: some runners find KT tape too heavy-duty and can be irritated by the glue backing. In this instance, and if you'd still like to tape, you might want to try Hypafix, which is a tape made from non-woven material with a polyester backing and a low-allergy adhesive. It is lighter, less heavy-duty and can often work just as well.

## Dress for success!

If you take anything away from this chapter, let it be this: you do not need to spend loads of money on kit. And with second-hand online stores such as Vinted or eBay so easily accessible, the availability of cost-effective second-hand/bought-but-not-worn options is endless – from trainers to tops, bum bags to backpacks, coats to hats. You can go crazy spending money on running kit but – if you have some of the above items, your trainers and a bra being the two most important – you will have all you need to start this joyful journey.

## CHAPTER 5

# All the feels

If you've tried running before and failed, you probably started off by running too fast.

If you've tried running before and hated every minute of it, you probably started off by running too fast.

If you've tried running before and got injured before you even really got going. Yep, you probably started off by running too fast.

Do you know what puts women who I have coached, or spoken to, off learning to run more than anything else? It's the thought of having to run fast. Faster than they ever have, want to, or believe they should. It's the thought of being left behind by a group they join because they believe, and maybe others even insinuated by their words and actions, that they are too slow.

(The other factor is safety, as I've already mentioned – but I dedicate an entire chapter to that later.)

If you have ever experienced any of the above, then you are far from alone. Please know this: how you feel both physically and mentally when you make the decision to start to run is what will keep you coming – or not coming – back.

We live in a 24/7, always-on world that sells us products and services that have been designed to tell us what we should eat, how we should move, what internal and external biological metrics we should track, when to wake up, when to go to sleep, etc. As a result, many of us have lost the ability to allow ourselves the time and space to tune into our bodies to understand what they are telling us and how we can respond to this. To read the cues that they give us of what feels, and doesn't feel, good.

Through learning to run with me, I want to help you tune into your body, and the cues it gives you, when learning to run. I want to empower you to block out the external influence of people, products and services that – even if promoted as 'being there to support your journey' – will take away from you listening to your gut instinct.

And I'm going to do that by sharing my advocacy for a form of training that is based on learning to understand how you feel during every running session I craft for you.

That form of training – of learning to run based on feel – is called rate of perceived exertion (RPE) training.

But first, there are a couple of important things I want to share.

> According to a study on runners participating in Couch to 5K programmes, 64.5 per cent of participants dropped out, with 74.6 per cent dropping out before the halfway point.

## Don't believe the hype

There are thousands of training plans that you can view online, loads of podcasts and couch to 5K apps that you can use for guidance and advice, and virtual and in-person running clubs and communities that you can join. Just type 'What pace should I start to run at?' into a search engine and prepare to be overwhelmed by the amount of information out there.

I'm guessing that some of you reading this book have tried one, or a few, of these, and it hasn't worked out for you. You're not alone.

In the many years that I have been running I've done it all. I've tried following training plans with running paces that are calculated based on my current 5K time. I've tried one-to-one coaching with people who had no idea how my hormone levels – as we will discuss in chapters 9 and 10 – affect how I run on any given day. I've tried running apps that ask me to predict a goal race finish time and, using that, prescribe paces for me to run at. I've tried running in groups that went faster than I could run because I was told, 'If you want to be faster, you've got to run with fast people.'

For a few years, at the start of my running career, when I wanted to get better but didn't know how, I hurt myself – both mentally and physically – testing all the above. I was running at paces that were not suitable, at effort levels that did not make me a stronger runner, and beating myself up because I wasn't getting any better. Why? Because that's what I read or was told I should do. If you want to achieve X then you need to train Y. And if you can't – do you even want it enough?

I was always good enough. You are good enough.

It was – and to an extent still is – the science that lets us down.

# Women are not small men

Running science has historically been biased towards men, with most studies often excluding or under-representing women. Why? Because we are seen as complex individuals when it comes to study. We are not as simple as men!

Among other things, we have been excluded because we have fluctuating hormone levels (e.g. the menstrual cycle), which can affect data analysis. We have been excluded because studies haven't focused on researching how to optimise training for our different menstrual cycles or in perimenopause and menopause – see chapter 10.

We have been excluded because studies fail to account for physical and biomechanical differences between women and men, leading to less – effective injury prevention protocols and rehabilitation strategies aimed at us. We are excluded because there are not enough of us in positions of influence and power – from elite athletes to coaches and researchers – which means this bias is further perpetuated.

Bethan Taylor-Swaine – a feminist sociologist of sport – says of the barriers that women face when learning to run: 'Sport has historically been male-dominated: it is a way to define and reinforce masculinity and the way that it privileges men in society more widely through demonstrations of strength, grit and endurance, to the exclusion of women.

'While we've come a long way, sport remains heavily coded as masculinity continues to be a way for men to assert their power and dominance in society.'

This issue – the gender bias in sports science – is one that over the years has gained more recognition. But still, to this day, there is not enough research conducted on us that can inform us appropriately and can be translated into meaningful resources that we can use, including things like running training plans, products and services.

In terms of research, the gender imbalance has led to massive gaps in the true understanding of how physiological, hormonal and biomechanical differences between women and men affect how we learn to run, our training and the risks associated with that.

All those years ago, I was good enough. It was the science informing everything I saw, touched and tasted associated with running and gender-biased science that wasn't. Well-meaning souls would say to me, 'But Sabs, the numbers don't lie!' But they do. Because those numbers (and by 'numbers' in the context of this chapter, I mean training paces) don't represent me. In fact, not only do they not represent me, I don't think they represent teenage girls, adult women, child-bearing women, menstrual women, perimenopausal and menopausal women, or ageing women either.

Bethan has this important point to add: 'It's also important to stress that context is often missing when people quote statistics on social media. It means we are often missing vital nuance. People's misunderstanding of data/research is a big one for the science communication community presently.'

So, how do we combat that? How do I enable you to truly 'find your feet' during the running journey you are about to go on, and feel joy in the process? Real joy that leads to consistency and healthy progression? Well, I am going to share with you a training protocol that will enable you to look for all you need 'inside you'. A system of running that will enable you to better trust yourself and what your body needs on any given day.

A way to listen to cues that your body gives you physically, biologically and mentally.

I want you to learn to trust your gut instinct through understanding, and working with, your rate of perceived exertion.

> **DEFINE 'EXERTION'**
>
> Physical or mental effort. 'She looked like she was really exerting herself during that run.'

## What is rate of perceived effort training?

The thing I love about RPE training – or, as I prefer to call it, 'feel'-based training – is that it is dictated entirely by *you* and how *you* feel on any given day.

How does every single run being a celebration of you sound? How does the idea of not one single run being classified as 'bad' sound? Good? Read on.

RPE training is a method that allows you to gauge your exercise intensity (in this case running intensity) based on how hard it feels for *you*. What so many running coaches love about this way of training is that it uses subjective cues like breathing, muscle fatigue, mental and emotional cues and overall effort to gauge training level – rather than relying solely on other factors such as pace, power or heart rate.

RPE training uses various scales to measure intensity. One of the best known is called the BORG Effort Scale. It's really easy to understand so, for beginners, it's the one I recommend. And it looks like this.

| RPE scale | Effort level | Activity |
|---|---|---|
| 0 | Rest | |
| 1 | Really easy | This might look like a walk. Breathing will be very light. You could sing if you wanted to. |
| 2 | Easy | This might look like a brisk walk, gentle run/walk or slow jog. You can talk in complete sentences. Breathing will be light. |
| 3 | Moderate | You are breathing a bit deeper. This would be a pace you could hold consistently for the required time. You can still hold a conversation, but sentences might be shorter. |
| 4 | Sort of hard | This might look like a longer period, or a slightly faster period, of running. It will feel a bit harder. You will breathe even deeper. It's comfortably uncomfortable. |
| 5 | Hard | This might look like a session where I ask you to run intervals or hill repeats. You are going to be working hard. You will only be able to utter a few words. |
| 6 | Hard + | You will be breathing even harder. Fewer words being uttered. |
| 7 | Really hard | Your breathing is deep and laboured. You will only be able to run for shorter bursts. |
| 8 | Really hard + | Very deep and very laboured breathing. No words. |
| 9 | Really, really hard | You will be giving it all you can. |
| 10 | Maximal | Maximum effort. |

Some women find it easier to think about a traffic-light system:

- Amber: RPE levels 1–2
- Green: RPE levels 3–4
- Red: RPE levels 5–10

To quell any fears you have right now, I want to state that on my training plan you will be spending most of your time, let's say 80 per cent of it, in the amber and green zones (1–4). You can now release that breath that you have been holding in! It's in those areas of training that you will find joy, consistency and, I hope, a love for running.

However, the red zones (5–10) are there for a reason. And the easiest way for me to explain that reason is for you to visualise something for me.

Close your eyes and imagine yourself standing inside a box.

1. Stretch your arms out to the side and imagine yourself touching the left- and right-hand sides of the box. That is where you are now. It is the size of your current box.
2. I want you to imagine walking to the right-hand side of the box and using your strength to push it (whether you push it with both hands or with your body is up to you!). As you push the right-hand side (go on, really lean against it) the box gets a bit bigger, with all four sides expanding outwards.
3. Now go back and stand in the centre of the box and straighten your arms out again. You can't touch the sides anymore, can you?
4. Walk forwards and, with both hands, push against the front. Go on, really push! Give it some welly! Your effort is causing the whole box to expand again. The box is now even bigger than it was before.

Every time we push ourselves, whether in running or in life – and science proves it – we grow. We grow mentally and physically. Whether we use brain training on puzzles like sudokus, crosswords and Wordle or spend some time in the red zone (RPE 5-plus) when learning to run, we grow.

To become more resilient as a runner, to become stronger, to be able to run for a little longer, you need to venture every now and then into the red zone. I want to show you that you do not have to fear it. On this journey of learning to run 5K I want you to know that, when I ask you to exert effort that challenges you to push against the sides of your current box (your current running ability), it's because it will help you build your new running ability.

Mixing up amber, green and red zones (RPE 1–10) is how I, as a coach, will train you to run from 0 to 5K. During this programme you will get comfortable being uncomfortable – in small and large ways – but always in a safe way because you will be listening to your body.

> **DON'T OVERTHINK IT!**
>
> 'Just don't overthink it, and do it. Yes, it's hard initially but it gets easier quickly and your future self will thank you. You will feel stronger; your mind will be clearer. The endorphins won't necessarily "fix" any mental health problems, but they will help you to cope. And please, don't compare yourself to others. Just be kind to yourself and your own body.'

# Cues

So, how do you start to tune into your body using RPE? How do you even begin to know whether you're working at the level I assign you? Here are some key things to think about when tuning into your body for effective understanding of your very own RPE.

### Take my breath away

As indicated in the table on p. 68, how you breathe closely correlates with how much effort you might be feeling and that I can tell – as a coach – you are putting in. For example, if I am out running with a woman on what is supposed to be a RPE 3-level run and she cannot hold a conversation with me, I know that she's working too hard. I'll encourage her to reduce to a slower-paced run, a walk/run or even a walk in order to be able to bring down her breathing rate.

And it's important for you to remember that your RPE 3–4 will be different to that of Shirley down the road or the woman on social media who can run fast and talk at the same time. Believe me, there is absolutely no point in comparing yourself to anyone else.

And what if I asked you to work at RPE 1–2? Well, that means you'd be breathing easily; it'd be barely noticeable. You'd be able to sing me a song if I asked you to. Hit RPE 7, though, and you'd be struggling to string a sentence together: three words might be all you can manage. At RPE 8–9? Silence is golden.

It'll take some practice, but if you truly tune in – understanding how your breath rate corresponds to RPE – it won't take long for you to be able to assess your RPE effectively.

> **SLOW DOWN!**
>
> 'Slow down and then slow down some more. That's my secret to falling in love with running in the beginning. If it feels hard, just slow down, even if it feels you could walk faster. Run with your head held high and proud. You are amazing.'

## Sweat rate

What happens to you physically is a key cue, too. With increased activity, you are going to sweat. We are hormonal beings, and our sweat rate will vary based on fluctuating hormone levels, the time of the month, the clothes we are wearing, the ambient temperature, etc. But sweat rate is a way that you can assess how hard you are working. Sweating a lot? You are probably nearing, or in, the red zone (5–10).

## Temperature

You are going to feel warmer. If you are in the luteal phase of your period, or perimenopause, you may feel warmer all the time (I know I do) but, also, it's a marker for how much effort you are putting in when running. You'll find you want to take off that jacket after a few minutes, and then your long-sleeved T-shirt. You'll also soon bin the leggings for shorts (I promise you!). And the more effort you put in, the hotter you will get. Your body's natural response to heating up is to cool itself down by releasing sweat (it interacts with air and cools the body). If you put in more effort, you heat up, and you sweat more.

## Feel your way

How does your body, your muscles in particular, feel? When we are walking, walk/running or running between RPE 2 and RPE 4 the stress on our bodies is lower. This can lead us, with practice, to feel like we could move at that pace – if we needed to – forever. For me, running in that wonderful green zone of RPE 3–4 is the sweet spot. You may hear it described as running 'in the zone' or 'running nirvana'. It's that physical feeling of being able to run in a way that is sustainable for us as individuals, that is joyful, that promotes consistency. Because our bodies *feel* good at this pace. Our muscles don't feel tight, there's no heaviness in our legs. We're in a flow state. But, of course, as we start to increase intensity – to move into the higher RPE levels – our bodies signal to us that there is more effort going on. Our muscles become tighter, it's harder to raise our knees with each step, we might start to feel that tingle, or burn, of our bodies not being able to clear lactate (waste product) from our muscles quickly enough. We might even find it difficult to stay tall. Notice everything. These signs are the cues that your effort level is increasing.

## Listen to your heart

When we are at rest and getting on with our day, we often don't hear our heartbeat. But I guarantee you, as you exert yourself up the RPE levels, you may hear it loud and clear – pounding in your ear, in your head. Increased heart rate is of course linked with RPE training, but I don't need you to run out and get a heart rate monitor to tell you that you are working harder. Your senses will feel it – especially your senses of hearing and touch (just feel your pulse in your wrist or neck).

## Energy requirements

When you are working at a lower RPE level your body will rely mostly on stored energy (in the form of carbohydrates that have been stored as glycogen in your muscles) and stored fat as your fuel. Have you ever heard of the fat-burning zone? Well, that zone is found in the low- to mid-RPE zones. You will find that, for most of your runs, you will not need to take a high-carbohydrate snack out with you (again, this is based on individual needs and whether you have fuelled well beforehand). However, when working at RPE 6-plus, you may feel you need quick-release energy in the form of a snack – an energy bar, a gel, some jelly beans – to get you through it. Why? Because you are demanding more of your body and it needs energy, and quickly, to fuel it. That's another clue to your RPE.

## Mental and emotional

You may be a total beginner or you might be returning to running after a significant break. At times, this journey is going to feel mentally and emotionally hard. Because you are juggling life, too. But I know you can do it. If I ask you to do a proportion of your run at something that feels like RPE 7, you may need to quite literally 'get your head in the game'. Higher-intensity runs will feel more challenging and you may well think, 'I can't do this.' On those days, the run may require you to really focus. To really dig deep and 'keep your why close by'.

## Reading the cues

All these cues, every one of them, come together to give you that central indicator of your individual perceived rate of perceived exertion. I can't tell you what that is, because you need to feel into it. The process starts with you trusting yourself, being guided by what your body tells you and interpreting that. It's the wonderful holistic combination of all the cues – physical, mental, emotional – that will aid your progression on this journey.

Some questions to ask yourself in order to check your RPE:

- Could I sing out loud if I wanted to? (RPE 1–2)
- Do I feel good and like I could go on like this for a while? (RPE 3–4)
- How much energy do I have to continue doing what is being asked of me? (A lot = RPE 1–4)
- Am I able to have a conversation? (RPE 1–4)
- Am I sweating a lot? (RPE 6+)
- Am I physically tired and is it affecting this run? (Yes = RPE 6-plus)

Asking questions like this to check in with yourself, maybe every five minutes, will keep you present in the moment, in your body and on the run. The answers your body gives you will inform that from-the-gut assessment of what is going on for you in terms of your own exertion.

This way of training works and, for women beginning their running journey, I believe is the best training protocol there is. It's the best way of understanding where you are on any given day, at any given time. Guided by you, for you.

> **JUST DO IT!**
>
> 'Just do it. The feeling you get at the end of a run is amazing. Never compare yourself to anyone else: it is your journey. There will always be people who are faster than you; that's life. But remember you are out there doing it! It will help you to find yourself a running group – in-person or virtual – where you'll receive the love and support you need in your journey.'

## Painting by numbers

People who run can, and do, fall into the trap of being obsessed by numbers. Early on in my journey this obsession almost stopped me running. Why? Because the numbers – from personal bests to race times, from paces that I was told I had to maintain to 'get faster' to numbers I was told I had to hit on the scale to be slimmer (which they said equated to faster) – became unreachable. They became unhealthy obsessions and, over time, sucked all the joy out of running for me.

I don't want that for you.

The RPE scale, and the levels associated with it, are a way for you to check in with yourself, to not compare yourself with others or beat yourself up. I share it with you so you can connect and understand where you are, from day to day, in terms of exertion levels when you are performing running sessions. And you know what, if you practise this consistently, one day you won't need to allocate a number to that feeling; you'll just know where you are. It's beautiful to run free.

I also want you to know that your numbers in terms of RPE levels will – because you are a complex masterpiece of a woman – change daily, weekly and monthly. It's natural! What may feel like an RPE 4 run one day might feel like an RPE 7 or 8 the next time you try the same run. Conversely, a run I ask you to do might look hard on paper (RPE 7) but, when you are doing it, doesn't feel as tough. In fact, you smash the run and feel like Wonder Woman! It's important for you to know that absolutely everything that happens in your life feeds into how you will feel on a run. From sleep to food, from menstrual cycle to perimenopause, from personal to professional stressors, everything has an impact. Running is not linear. This is another reason why this form of feel-based training works. Because whether a RPE 4 means a comfortable run one day and a walk the next, it's OK. You are doing what I have asked you to do and are responding in the moment.

And you are all I care about. You are not a number.

I will caveat this by saying that I know that some of you will want to run with a watch, for personal or medical reasons, and that is OK. All I would say is to please trust yourself and the progress you are making over the statistics on a watch.

Feel the fear and do it anyway!

CHAPTER 6

# Walk this way

A few weeks ago I was at a community running event. It was a 5K run around the streets of Wembley and was pitched as a 'social' run. A 'social' run usually means the speed is at a 'comfortable pace'. This is also known as an 'aerobic' or 'forever' pace or – when thinking about RPE – the pace of a green run. To simplify it even more, it's a pace that means that you can hold a conversation with another person or, if you should feel so inclined (and I have many times), with yourself or the dog.

However, during this run, it became quickly apparent that the pace being set was far from social. In fact, for some participants, it was so challenging that they could only speak in hurried three-word sentences. As a coach, it is my job to understand what is happening to the runners around me by visually and verbally monitoring them.

Laboured breathing? Too fast. Not able to hold a conversation? Too fast. My clients asking me open-ended questions because they don't want to talk? Yes, you've guessed it – they are running too fast! All of these things are signs to me that they need to slow down.

Even though I wasn't being paid to be a run leader that day, I felt it was my moral duty to monitor the situation. I started talking to a woman who I could see was struggling to keep up. To allow her some breathing space, I non-verbally helped her adjust her pace by providing physical cues. I ran in step with her and then slowed down my pace, which, in turn, caused her to slow down, too. I then conveyed that I was going to take a small walk break so that I'd be 'ready for the final push', which she welcomed enthusiastically. But, as we were walking – and people were passing us – she said, 'I feel like a bit of a fraud because we should be running like the others, shouldn't we?'

And there, right there, in that question, is one of the biggest misconceptions about running that there is. That to be a runner, you must run consistently. That to be able to say you have run 5K or 10K or a half marathon or a marathon and more, you must run the whole thing.

This is not true. You do not.

Walking during a run, whether for pleasure, recovery, as part of a run/walk protocol or just because you want to, is probably one of the single most important things that you can do as a runner.

Walking makes you a more mentally and physically resilient runner. Walking allows you to reset, recover and go again. It is a tool in running that is practised and utilised by beginners, keen amateurs and top-level athletes across road, trail, fell and mountain running.

Walking is part of running.

> **MY 5K AND ME**
>
> 'I thought I was too old to start running but, when I looked at the photo, I saw a woman who looked the same age as me so it spurred me on to give it a try. The journey was hard at times: I am not as fast as some of the others, but the ability to walk as part of my running was the option I needed to stay consistent. It got me to the end of my 10-week programme and I got my 5K medal (that my coach made). I am so glad I took the step to decide to try.'

## Breaking down barriers

The running industry has a lot of work to do when it comes to breaking down barriers in running. And, as someone who understands the power of words, I know that quite a few of the barriers to women accessing this activity lie in the terminology used.

Even the word 'run' can be off-putting, can't it? Countless women – and it *is* mostly women – have said to me, 'How can I say I have been on a run if I have walked a quarter of it?' 'How can I claim to be a runner, if I haven't run the whole way?'

Some women report back that other people (usually men) have commented on how they choose to move. 'C'mon love, it's called a trail run, not a trail walk.'

How can you claim you are a runner? Because YOU can.

If you set out to run – even if you only run a tenth of it – you are a runner. And it's walking that is a key ingredient to making you a stronger, more efficient runner. By using the information I am going to share with you below – and intentionally putting it into practice when you are running – I invite you to challenge anyone who says otherwise. And I mean anyone – whether family, friends or strangers. Anyone who questions a runner who chooses to walk as part of their run, needs to be fact-checked.

## It wasn't made for us – we must claim it!

I want you to remember that the activity of running has, until relatively recent times, been a male-dominated, male-marketed sport. And, in some cases – even though there has been a shift towards more studies and marketing campaigns aimed at increasing female inclusion in running – it still is.

> From the 1920s to the 1960s women were often barred from long-distance running events due to outdated beliefs about their physical limitations. It was at the 1960 Olympic Games in Rome that the International Olympic Committee (IOC) started to allow women to compete in races longer than 800 metres.

The science used to create the hundreds of thousands of training plans that you can find online are mostly based on research on men. The many running products available, including trainers, have usually been created and sold based on the physiology of men. Events that are marketed as 'inclusive for all' commonly base their event cut-off times on the times of – yes, you've guessed it – men.

But we can change things. Through our intentional actions to claim running as our own, women like you and me are being the change we need to see – and want future generations to see. But in order to do that we have to reframe, first for ourselves and then for others, what running is.

And running includes walking.

> **'I WAS ALWAYS RUNNING; I JUST DIDN'T KNOW IT.'**
>
> Hillary Gerardi is an elite athlete who, in 2023, recorded the fastest known time (FKT) from Chamonix, France, to the summit of Mont Blanc (4,806 metres/15,767 feet) and back. She completed this running challenge in 7.25 hours. She walked (power hiked) as well as ran.
>
> She explained: 'I worked in mountain huts when I was in university, and I loved it. I loved hiking. I loved maps. I loved imagining itineraries. I didn't identify what I did as running because I thought that with running, you had to be running the whole time. I didn't do trail "races", but I was trail running; I just didn't call it that. Admittedly, I thought running was boring. I thought it was lame. I was a hiker. I didn't identify as a runner for a long time.
>
> 'I personally feel that we have a vocabulary problem in trail running because if you say somebody is not running, it comes off as if it's a value judgement. I was talking to a friend who had done a really long race, and I was totally in awe. But if you look at the statistics, he was probably hiking 99 per cent of the time. I said as much, and his response was, "No, I ran it!" And I was like, "Hey, I'm not judging."'

## And I would walk 500 miles . . .

And that's a big part of the problem – the fear of being judged. Of being seen as 'less than' if we walk during a run. But Hillary isn't less than, is she? She ran the women's fastest known time!

Go to *any* running event, or race, and you will see people walking. Some of them will not have planned for it, some of them will have done, and some of them – due to injury – will have to. But, I guarantee you, you will see people walking.

> ### PARKWALK
>
> You've probably heard of the 5K running phenomenon called Parkrun, the global event that engages over 340,000 people weekly at 2,000-plus locations around the world. Every Saturday and Sunday people take part in a free, weekly, timed 5K run. In October 2022, to cater for people who might find running intimidating, the company launched Parkwalk. This event co-exists with weekly Parkruns and aims to make the event more inclusive and accessible for everyone, regardless of fitness level.

The training plan – which will take you from couch to 5K – that I have designed for you in the Miles and Smiles chapter on page 212 incorporates walking. Let's look at why walking is so important in the journey to making you a consistent, stronger and more resilient runner.

## Walk to . . . support the progression of your running practice

Every training plan that I have ever followed since I started running has included walking as a key component. This might have been walking for recovery or power hiking – or, as I call it, 'walking with purpose' – uphill, downhill or on the flat.

Each session I have planned for you includes walking. And if you ignore the walking that I have incorporated, then my experience as a coach shows that it is highly likely you will not complete the 10-week plan. Walking allows beginners, or those returning to running after a break, to ease into the activity without overexerting themselves. In my plans, walking is used to recover and as part of interval training (more on that on pp. 82 and 100). All sessions have been designed to improve your moving speed (pace) and the amount of time you are on your feet (endurance).

It's important that you know that all training plans are, or certainly should be, designed around something called 'progressive overload'. What that means, in simple terms, is that over a specific time period or 'micro-phase' (say, four weeks) your body will experience a cycle of managed progression, overload and recovery. That cycle, if followed correctly, will lead to your body adapting to the demands placed upon it, which, in turn, will make you a stronger runner. You will become a runner who can move a little bit more quickly, for a little bit longer.

## Walk to . . . maintain a comfortable heart rate

Most people who say they 'hate running' probably run too fast. Yep, you got it: they haven't walked enough. I always monitor whether the people I coach are working at a level that ensures that their heart is working aerobically (zone 2). I like to hear them have a full conversation while they are training. If that means they must walk, so be it.

And how does someone who is brand new to the activity of running ensure that they – their heart – are not working too hard? They take walk breaks.

### WHAT IS ZONE 2 HEART RATE (HR) TRAINING?

It refers to whether you are exercising at a specific intensity within your *aerobic* heart rate zone. This means that you are working at a level of effort in which your body is efficiently using oxygen to produce energy and primarily burning fat as fuel. Want to know what yours is? Well, it's typically 60–70 per cent of your maximum heart rate (MHR), measured in beats per minute (BPM).

To calculate your zone 2 range, use this equation:
(220 – your age) x 0.6 = lower end of zone 2 HR
(220 – your age) x 0.7 = upper end of zone 2 HR

For example:

For a 38-year-old woman: (220 − 38) x 0.6 = 109.2. (220 − 38) x 0.7 = 127.4. Therefore the zone 2 HR range would be 109 to 127 BPM.

For a 48-year-old woman: (220 − 48) x 0.6 = 103.2. (220 − 48) x 0.7 = 120.4. Therefore the zone 2 HR range would be between 103 and 120 BPM.

Well-respected running coach Steve Magness says: 'When people recommend zone 2 training for the general population, for most it should mean to go for a walk. I'd hate running if every day it felt hard or moderately hard (RPE 5–10/red).

'Hard workouts are enjoyable because they are occasional. They allow you to challenge yourself and, mostly, succeed. If they are every day, they demoralise and demotivate. What's the easy pace for someone trying to exercise? Walking.'

## Walk to . . . improve form and breathing

Incorporating walking intervals gives you a chance to regroup 'on the run' and check in on how you feel physically and mentally. As we move through each week's sessions you will see that – as you start to be on your feet for longer – you will tire. I see this energy depletion physically in women when their shoulders start to droop forwards, their back starts to hunch, they look down (rather than ahead) and they start to scuff their feet due to not lifting their knees high enough. All of these are signs that your form is slipping. Taking walk breaks will give you a chance to address that. A chance to remember to pull your shoulders back, engage your core muscles and release tension by shaking out your arms. And to focus on controlling your breathing. To take some deep breaths in for three counts and out for four counts. To take back control of your oxygen uptake. To remember that you are OK, that you are safe, and that this is part of the process.

## Walk to . . . recover on the move

It's important to recover while on the move, but we don't want to stop, so we walk. By incorporating walking into your runs, you are encouraging newly oxygenated blood to flow to your muscles, which in turn helps to clear lactic acid and reduce associated feelings of soreness. Allowing this process to take place is essential for you to be able to progress as a runner and practise your running consistently.

## Walk to . . . go longer

My aim is to take you from couch to 5K. Each week I will increase the amount of time you are on your feet and the proportion of that time that is spent running. Utilising walking as part of the weekly plan will allow me to subtly inch up your overall running session time, which in turn will build your endurance without overexerting you. I want you to finish each session feeling strong, not broken. Feeling fabulous, not fried. Walking gives you that.

## Walk to . . . reduce injury

Guess how much the force exerted on your body is when running? It's two and a half to three times your bodyweight with *each stride*. When it comes to joints, research shows that the knee joint alone experiences compressive forces up to eight times your bodyweight on each stride. That's a lot, eh? So, take off some of that load during a run, and walk. By doing this you'll not only reduce the overall force exerted on your body, but you'll also find yourself better able to tune into anything else that may be going on. I don't want you to *battle* through your running sessions. Learning to run is not supposed to be a physical and mental war. My own experience has taught me that it is often in those walk breaks, when I am able to really tune into my body, that I become aware of any areas of tightness, a niggle or pain. It's in the walking that I become aware that something does not feel right and I can either address it there and then or take action, post-run, to get further advice.

Our bodies are a walking, talking encyclopaedia of all physical and mental trauma – no matter how large or small – that we have experienced in our lives. As I will cover in chapter 11, niggles and running injuries often come about because of what we have experienced historically and how we live our lives daily.

## Walk to . . . reduce fatigue post run

My aim is for you to finish your run feeling good, not spent. Feeling like, if you had to, you could do a little bit more. I do not want you to cross the threshold of your home only for your legs to give way and for you to be unable to function as a normal human being for the day(s) ahead.

There is a time and place for *that* type of running exertion and it's not in this book!

Walking during your run will make you feel much less fatigued both during and post run. Why post run? By reducing your perceived exertion – by walking – during your run your body has less biological damage to repair afterwards. Therefore, the energy needed to 'recover' is lessened and – hey presto – you have more energy to get on with your day and are ready to head into the next session feeling good, because you haven't smashed yourself during your run. You have managed your training in a way that is effective and efficient. No post-run 'bonk' for you.

> ### BONKING
>
> To 'bonk' or 'hit a wall' is a term used in running when you, quite simply, don't have enough available energy to power what is being asked of your body. You have used up all your available glycogen (energy source) and your body isn't producing the amount you need, quickly enough, from its fat stores. You start to feel weak and can experience heavy legs and negative mindset. You have bonked. This can happen to people during the run and in the immediate recovery time after. As I discuss in chapter 12, refuelling post run is important.

## Walk to . . . chunk the run

Whether you are running one mile or a hundred miles, chunking is your friend. It refers to cutting your run up into manageable sections. The start and end of a 'chunk' is determined by the action you take. In this case, walking. When it comes to increasing your mental stamina, there is power in you knowing, before going on a run, that you will be moving for a certain amount of time – or distance – before you get a walk break. Chunking can help make your running practice feel manageable and less daunting. I often say to the women I coach that 'the thought of a run can often stop us lacing up our shoes and getting out of the door' – and this is where chunking helps. I've experienced my fair share of thinking, 'Oh god, I don't think I can *run* for that distance today.' So, believe me, your mental stamina will benefit from using walking to keep you motivated enough to have a go at a session even on those days when it feels harder to venture outside.

## Walk to . . . increase running joy

I'm all about the joy. I almost called this book *RunJoy* because that is what I want women to experience when learning to run solo or in a community. I want you to enjoy it. I really do. I know that may seem like me asking a lot. And I know that, depending on our lives, our hormones and our past and present experiences, there will be days when you run and you don't feel joy all the way. But I do believe that walking is a conduit to running joy. Taking time to walk helps keep us present on the run. It can stop running being a chore because you know that you are going to get the chance to tune into your body, to control your breathing, to check in. There is so much enjoyment to be had through moving our bodies in this way and, sometimes, we must slow down and smell the roses in order to remember why we are out here doing this, today. Walking gifts us presence.

## Walk to . . . keep it social

There's an African proverb that says: 'If you want to go fast, go alone. If you want to go far, go together.' In the years that I have been training women to run, there is one thing that has worked during the sessions to cultivate community and connection and to strengthen the 'no person is left behind' ethos that I strongly advocate. Yep, it's walking. When we qualify, run coaches are taught how to keep mixed-ability groups together and a key tactic is to walk. The most connected running groups that I have coached, and been a member of, dictate their run paces as being 'as fast as the slowest person'. This protocol means that faster runners can still run at the pace they want to but they must 'loop back', meaning a coach like me can instigate walk breaks when everyone is together. Ultimately this means that everyone gets what they want out of a session, but the group is connected.

> ### JEFFING!
>
> It's not just me who believes in the power of walking to go faster and further. There's a massive global community of runners who, from 5K to long-distance running, use a run–walk–run method described by Jeff Galloway – an Olympian and renowned running coach. His technique involves alternating running and walking to complete runs of all distances. For example, a beginner might follow a 1:1 run/walk strategy (for instance, running for one minute, walking for one minute) while a marathon runner might employ a 4:1 ratio. Among its many other benefits, Jeffing promotes inclusivity, making it a much-loved way to train.

> ### RUN/WALK KEEPS RUNNING FUN
>
> 'Recovering from an injury introduced me to the run/walk method and it's been a total game-changer. What started as a recovery tool has now become a key strategy for me to use during most of my longer-distance events. Playing around with the run/walk ratios keeps running fun and interesting. Also, running the flats while walking the hills ensures I've always got energy left in the tank!'

Remember the woman earlier in the chapter who said she 'felt like a fraud' when she was walking during the 5K 'social' run? What do you think I told her? Well, not *all* of the above, but certainly the most salient points about the benefits of walking on the run. After our walk break we did eventually start running again and – due to the availability of energy – we were able to run the last 100 metres to the finish line much faster. She, and I, finished feeing like strong, powerful women, joyful women, women who had connected through choosing to walk on the run.

Were we runners? I'll leave you to answer that!

## CHAPTER 7

# Mounds of opportunity

There's an important truth that I want you to know when learning to run. A truth that, if you are reading this, I want you to prepare yourself for, because there is no getting away from it. You cannot hide from it. Well, actually, there is a way to hide from it but, if you do, your running will be boring – and the last thing I want is for you to be bored on the run. I want your running journey to offer you *mounds of opportunity*.

And by 'mounds of opportunity', I mean *hills*.

If you run, you will come across hills. And, as someone who runs, you will have to decide if you deviate around them and stay low, or face them head-on with the knowledge they are a thing to become familiar with, not fear. Hills are something that will make you a stronger, more resilient runner.

'Hills are my friend' is a mantra I use.

So, how do you become friends with something that, at the start of your running journey, you may fear?

Making friends with hills starts here.

What stops women running hills?

- 'I won't be able to make it to the top.'
- 'Everyone else is faster than me.'
- 'I can barely walk a hill, never mind run it.'
- 'Just looking at a hill makes me feel anxious.'
- 'It's already hard enough to run. Why make it harder?'
- 'I'm not sure how to?'

# Feel the fear and do it anyway

Every single time I stand in front of a new group of women who are learning to run 5K and I mention the words 'hill running', their eyes widen, mouths drop open and they often take a physical step back from me, as if I have burned them, as if stepping away will make what I have suggested less real.

I was the same when I learned to run. I did all I could to *not* run up hills. That involved me sticking to flat roads and the canal towpath because, you know, just running on these was exhausting enough! Why would I add another layer of difficulty?

But it was much more than that. I feared hills because of what they might *do* to me. And by that I meant how exhausted they might make me. I feared that I might not make it – even if I had to take walk breaks – to the top. That I might have a panic attack due to the overexertion of it. And, also, I didn't see any other female runners who looked like me running up hills. I didn't want to fail and look stupid for even trying.

So, what business did I have trying to run up hills? Why do it?

Because it matters. Because embracing hills – or mounds of opportunity – is one of the best things you can do to add variety to your running, to become a more resilient runner and to get some of the best running rewards that there are – those being a sense of accomplishment and a new perspective.

> **RUN/WALK ENABLES GREATER ACCESS**
>
> 'Having the confidence to run and walk hills has allowed me to extend my range of running options. I love being able to take my trainers onto the trails, as it gives me even greater access to the outdoors. There's nothing like that joyful sense of accomplishment when I reach a summit, and then the reward of flying back down it.'

# Pick a hill

I am fortunate in that I live in a hilly area of the United Kingdom so, when it comes to finding hills to practise running on, I have a lot of variety. From short, sharp inclines to gentle rolling hills, and from grassy mounds to more challenging stony terrain, whatever I want, I can get. But at the beginning of my running journey, it wasn't these hills I chose as my target to get up. The hill I chose was one that I used to drive the kids up to school every day (and sometimes I'd walk it with them too, but not often, as they'd complain about it). It was the same hill that I used to walk up as a kid with my mum and sister, and as a teenager on my way back from my Saturday job. The hill I chose had meaning to me because, through all those years, I never once imagined I'd try to run up it.

Do you have a hill like that? One local to you that is more than just 'a hill'. A hill that, if you were to run to the top of it, would be a massive achievement and would make you feel, quite literally, 'on top of the world'? Because never in your wildest dreams did you believe you could get to the top of it. Then that's your hill! I want you to make a note of it, right now. Write the name of that hill down either on a piece of paper or in the notes section of your phone. Write this: 'I choose to run to the top of [insert hill here]. This will be my mound of opportunity.'

You've taken the first important step in learning how to run hills. You've thought about a hill. You have associated it with you and running, and you have committed it to paper. Now, let's get into the why.

> **QUEEN OF THE WORLD**
>
> 'There is no better feeling than getting to the top of a hill at sunrise or sunset knowing my body – and mine alone – got me there. I feel powerful, I feel strong, I am the queen of the world!'

# Why run hills?

I am a stronger runner physically and mentally due to incorporating hills into my monthly running practice, as are the women I coach. And you will be, too. Yes, you will be challenged, no doubt about it. But every hill is an opportunity and, in terms of getting bang for your buck from your training, hills are the gift that keeps on giving.

Some of the benefits of incorporating them into your running practice include:

**Strength gains** – Hill running will cause you to engage your gluteal muscles (bum), hamstrings, calves and core muscles much more than running on the flat will. In this sense, it's a form of moving resistance training as you'll be working against gravity, therefore strengthening key muscle groups used for running without the need for weights. Winner, winner, chicken dinner!

**High-intensity interval training (HIIT)** – Adding hills into your running will elevate your heart rate more quickly than running on the flat. Hill running, especially repetitions – which allow for recovery between each rep – is a form of HIIT that will enhance your endurance and cardiovascular health by increasing the amount of oxygen your body can use (your $VO_2$ max), strengthening your heart, which will enable it to pump blood more efficiently and improve your recovery.

**It'll make you stronger and faster on the flat** – It takes more effort to propel yourself uphill. For each step you take, you will be developing explosive (plyometric) strength and power in your legs, and you will see this translate to how you run on the flat (over time, it will feel easier).

**Better running form** – If practised correctly, and I'll talk about this more below, running uphill will encourage you to have better posture, a stronger knee drive and a more efficient arm swing, which will translate to better overall running form.

**Lower impact** – Running uphill is lower impact than downhill and flat running.

**Mental resilience** – Those women who incorporate hill running into their practice know, and rave about, the mental resilience it gives them. There is no better feeling than knowing that your body can conquer hills. My experience is that this knowledge can give you the confidence to push past other hard things in your running journey, and life, too.

**Variety is the spice of life** – Hills are the icing on your running cake. They are the ingredient that you never thought you needed but, when added, give your training that certain kick.

**The views** – My favourite running spot is a location near where I live. The climb can seem brutal but once I get there the view of the surrounding countryside that I am rewarded with – and that stretches out far and wide in front of me – is the stuff of dreams. Every single time I run there I feel powerful, I feel alive, I thank God that running gave me the ability to do this. And I want that for you, too.

## Small steps, big strides

I do not expect you to run consistently uphill from the get-go. Hell no! I am not a sadist. Learning to run uphill, and downhill, too, is a process. And, because uphill running is just *a part* of my plan to get you to run 5K your way – not the main goal – you will be starting small. You can breathe a sigh of relief!

Of course, your hill-running practice will include walking because – as we discussed in chapter 6 – a key part of running *is* walking. For hill-running practice, that might look like chunking an uphill session (run, walk, run, walk). It might look like the recovery (downhill) section of a set of hill intervals or, if on a longer endurance run, it might look like power hiking up the inclines.

> **FIND YOUR INNER CHILD**
>
> 'I love the challenge of hills. They allow me to get into a different rhythm on a run, which makes it more interesting! Plus, I love running downhill! I put my arms out like a plane and enjoy those moments of play.'

# Hill running dos and don'ts

I've run a shed load of hills – still do – and have coached many women to not only run them but to *love* running them. To actively seek them out. Below are some practical steps that I'd advise you to remember when learning to run hills.

## Warm-up and mobility

Always spend 5–10 minutes warming up. The warm-up should, ideally, be done on the flat because the aim is to warm up your muscles for the work they will soon be doing and to gently increase your heart rate. The warm-up is *part of* the session, not the main event, so it needs to be treated as such. It's a time to prepare your body, and mind, for what is to come. Mobilisation, as you will see in the Miles and Smiles chapter on page 212, is also a must. When it comes to hills, there are some specific mobilisation exercises I would advise you employ, including:

# LEG SWINGS

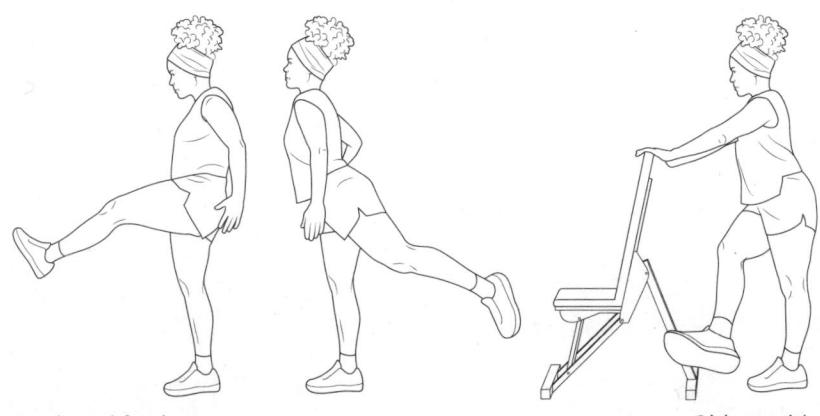

Back and forth                                        Side to side

- **Leg swings (back and forth)** – Stand side-on next to something upright, such as a wall, for support. Stand tall and engage your core (suck in your tummy). Swing your outside leg (the one furthest from the wall) forwards and backwards, keeping it as straight as you can. Control the movement and keep your hips facing forwards. Don't *throw* your legs back and forth. As you are swinging the leg, there will be a tendency for your hips to want rotate outwards. Really concentrate on keeping them facing forwards. Repeat 10 times and then change position and switch legs.

- **Leg swings (side to side)** – Stand face-on next to something upright, such as a wall or the back of a chair as pictured, for support. Support your upper body using straightened arms to lean against it. Pick a leg and swing it out to the side and then back in so that it crosses your other leg (in front of it). Keep the swinging leg as straight as possible. Repeat 10 times and then switch legs.

**Benefit: Why am I doing this?** It opens your hips and improves flexibility in your hamstrings and hip flexors.

## WALKING LUNGES WITH TORSO TWIST

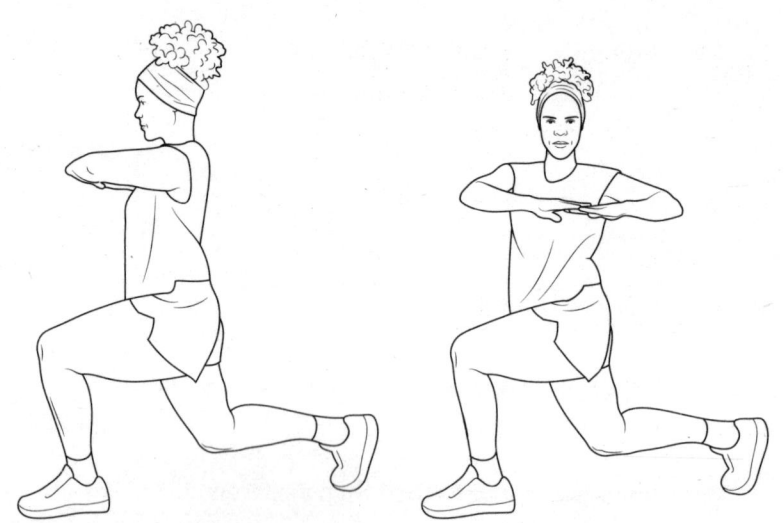

Stand tall, core engaged. Step one foot forwards so the leg bends into a lunge position. To achieve the correct position when in the lunge, the aim is for your knee to be sitting directly over your ankle and your lower leg to be at a 90-degree angle to your upper leg. When you are in this position, clasp your hands in front of you and twist your torso (upper body), as far as you are able, to the same side as the forward-lunging leg. Once complete, bring the torso back to centre, step back and repeat on the other side. Repeat 10 times.

**Why am I doing this?** It increases mobility in your hips, quads and lower back while activating your core.

## HIGH KNEES

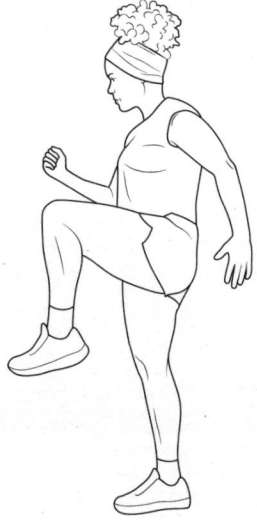

Jog on the spot, bringing your knees as far up towards hip height as you can. Pump your arms back and forth at the same time. Repeat this action for approximately 20 seconds.

**Why am I doing this?** It activates your hip flexors and improves your knee drive, which is crucial for uphill running.

# BUTT KICKS

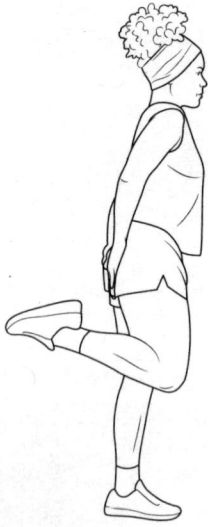

Jog on the spot, bringing your heels up towards your glutes (bum) as far as you can. I tend to place my hands on top of my glutes (palms facing outwards). This stabilises me and give my heels something to aim for. Repeat for approximately 20 seconds.

**Why am I doing this?** It loosens up the quads and improves hamstring flexibility.

## HEEL-TO-TOE WALKS

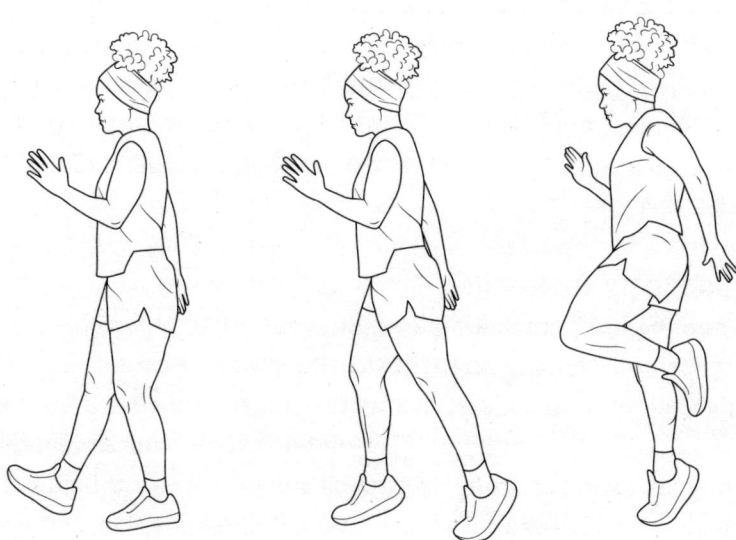

Walk forwards, rolling your foot from the back edge of your heel to the tip of your toes with each step. When you reach your toe, aim to fully extend your ankle (rise on to your tiptoes) and then repeat on the other side. Repeat 10 times.

**Why am I doing this?** It improves ankle mobility and strengthens the calves.

# Hill-running technique for beginners

How you run up, and down, a hill is different from how you run on the flat. It will take some time for you to get used to hill running because, naturally, your body will want to do the things you've been doing for years when ascending hills (staying low to the ground, looking down at your feet, hunching your shoulders). With practice, you will get there. Here are some top tips to set you off:

## Lean slightly forwards

Lean into the hill from your ankles, not your waist. This ankle lean will allow your body to stay aligned with the gradient of the hill you are looking to climb, and it will give gravity the best chance to assist you on the up. Those new to running hills tend to hunch their shoulders and bend too far forwards from the hips. It might feel like this is the best way to get up a hill (to almost resume a crawling position) but it's not. Think about it: if you hunch your shoulders and bend forwards all you are really doing is restricting your lung capacity. We don't want that. We want your lungs to have as much room to take on board as much oxygen as possible. So, stay tall.

## Shorten your stride

Take quicker, shorter steps. Running this way might, at times, feel like you are running on the spot but – I guarantee you – shortening your stride will help you to pick off that hill while ensuring efficient running technique and use of energy and maintaining uphill momentum. Taking long strides (because you think you'll get up the hill more quickly) will make the climb feel harder. I have been called 'twinkle toes' for my quicker, shorter uphill strides.

## Cadence

As discussed in chapter 3, cadence refers to the amount of times, normally per minute, that your feet hit the ground (steps per minute – SPM). When hill running, we are looking for a faster step turnover than when running on the flat.

> Between 160 and 180 steps per minute (SPM) is the range for easy/moderate runs. SPM will increase for hill running – due to faster, shorter steps.

## Engage your arms

Drive your arms forwards and back, keeping them parallel to each other as they move. Really try to not cross your arms in front of your body as that will impact on your technique, stability through the core and cause energy leakage (*see* p. 34). When it comes to hill running, the legs will do what the arms do. Coax your legs into moving uphill by pumping those arms back and forth like pistons. The steeper the incline, the more arm movement you may need. Another tip is to consciously remember to relax your hands. Don't clench your fists. It might help to imagine you are holding a delicate object like a crisp, a feather or an egg between your fingers and thumb with the gentlest grip.

### THE INVISIBLE RED ROPE

A visualisation trick that works for my runners when going uphill is to imagine a red rope on either side of you. With each swing of your arms, imagine you are pulling on that rope to haul yourself further uphill. You can even sync your hand movements to replicate what it would feel like to pull those parallel ropes. Try it: it might give you the extra pull that you need.

## Keep your gaze forwards

Look a few metres ahead of you. This will help you to maintain the required posture and balance. We can tend to look down when we are running uphill (often because looking up at where we are going can seem overwhelming). I am not asking you to look to the top of the hill, as that might throw your balance and posture off: just gaze ahead at what's directly in front of, not below, you.

## Avoid heavy heel striking

Try to avoid landing heavily into your heels when running uphill. A lighter landing, either on your forefoot or midfoot, can help you maintain momentum and reduce stressful impact. The power in each step you take comes mostly from your calves, hamstrings, glutes and quads, so intentionally think about them. I ask my runners to repeat out loud or silently 'calf, butt, calf, butt' with every set of four steps they take. It takes their mind off the job at hand and creates that connection between mind and muscle.

## Don't forget to breathe

This one seems obvious. I know, right? But sometimes we become so overwhelmed at the thought of a session, or while we are in it, that we forget to breathe rhythmically, or altogether, for too long a period. To get the most out of your hill-running practice it's important to try to breathe deeply and rhythmically to keep that oxygen flowing. If it helps, you can even try syncing your breathing with your steps to maintain a steady rhythm, but not to the point where it feels you are hyperventilating. Maybe try breathing in for three steps and out for three steps. The fun lies in experimenting and finding a rhythm that works for you.

## Run/walk intervals

Now, you know how important walking is to running. Well, its use in learning how to hill run effectively is no different. In my plan in the Miles and Smiles chapter on page 212 you will see that I use a run/walk strategy to help you break down or pick off your hill of choice using different time blocks. So, for example, I might ask you to run up a hill for 20 seconds and walk back down it at a pace that means you feel adequately recovered before starting the next repetition. Every time I ask you to do this run – either as part of the same session or as a new session – you will gently increase the time that you run uphill and take the recovery that you feel you need on the downhill. In another session I might ask you to 'pick off' a hill. This means that, although your end game is to get to the top, you will get there by picking a place on the hill that you feel you can run to. Once you hit that mark you will take time for a slower walk recovery (uphill) before picking the next place you will run to. Before you know it, you'll be at the top of the hill. All the best hill runners in the world use training sessions like this, and more, to hone their hill- and mountain-running skills. What works for them can work for you, too.

## Control your effort

Of course, hill running is going to feel challenging, as it should. If it were easy, everyone would do it. But please bear in mind that there's a big difference between a pace at which you are seeking to run a hill being challenging and it being unmanageable. Throughout this book we are focusing on manageable running. As we discussed in chapter 5, your pace – with hill running in particular – should be based on how you *feel*, not what others are doing or what externally prescribed numbers on an app tell you. It's about tuning into your body during your hill runs and using that indicator system we discussed on p. 73 as a guide. So, for example, using the traffic light indicator I might ask you to aim for a RPE 5–6/red level for the 'effort' section of a hill-repeats run. This would feel like a moderate-to-hard effort, but you could manage it. When learning to run hills your focus is not on running fast but being consistent. You should focus on getting to the end of the run feeling a sense of achievement, not failure. Getting your RPE right is key to that.

My friend Keri Wallace runs Girls on Hills – a women's trail running company that operates out of Glencoe, in Scotland. She has some great insights when it comes to running up and down hills!

### KEEP IT CONSISTENT

Keri: 'I often tell my runners to aim for a consistent effort level on undulating terrain, whether running on the flat or up hills. This is especially true for longer efforts – i.e. when you reach a hill, your cadence increases, and pace decreases, but the overall effort should be similar so that you can continue running when you reach the top (rather than having to stop and recover to pay back oxygen debt accrued by pushing too hard).'

## Recover well

Always allow yourself to recover well when you are practising hill running. I encourage you, as a beginner, to walk your recovery sections. Focus on intentionally slowing down your pace, take deep breaths, check in on your body, and ready the mind to go again. Walking your recovery will allow you the time and space to do that. It will also ensure that you are reducing the impact on your joints and muscles. If you in time decide to recover on a downhill at a jog, avoid overstriding and slamming your feet into the ground. There are more tips on downhill running below.

## Top of the world

If you follow the advice above and my plan then by the end of 10 weeks you will feel so much more confident when incorporating hills into your running sessions. I promise. To remain positive – and consistent – I really want you to celebrate each small milestone, because every one of them is a win. It might be that, on one session, you ran further up your hill than before or, in another session, you finished an extra hill repeat. Take a bow, girlfriend! You are a hill-running queen and should be celebrated as one! High fives all round.

> **SLOW AND STEADY WINS THE DAY**
>
> Anyone who has read the fable about the tortoise and the hare will understand the power of persistence and consistency to reach the finish line. When it comes to running up and down hills, it's important to manage your effort level. Because, over the weeks, step-by-step, you will improve. Be more tortoise!

> **SEE THE GOOD IN HILLS**
>
> 'I don't particularly enjoy hills, but I live in a very hilly city, so they are unavoidable. However, what I do enjoy is the way they force me to slow down. To think about my energy expenditure and my form. I also like the overall health benefits I feel they give me.'

# What to do when it's all going downhill

So, now you know the dos and don'ts of how to get your body uphill effectively, what do you do when you want to go downhill? Depending on the level you are at, and the experiences that you may have had, the speed at which you will feel comfortable descending will vary. I've had some falls, which have meant that – especially on more rocky ground – I can resemble a baby reindeer on ice when trying to run downhill. I can get so fearful of falling on the downhill sections that my form can go to pot because I'm anxious.

The way that you tackle a downhill not only depends on the terrain beneath your feet – is it concrete, grassy, rocky, muddy? – but also the steepness of the hill that you are descending. Running downhill requires control and concentration to not only get down safely, but also to avoid excessive overload on your muscles and joints.

> **ONE SMALL STEP AT A TIME**
>
> Keri: 'You want to keep your stride short and your steps nimble. It's about staying loose and being light on your feet – working "with" and not "against" gravity. Many women tend to look down at their feet but that's not necessarily the best place to focus. I encourage the people we coach to look further ahead of them – the place where they will next place their feet. What obstacles can you see? Where is best to land? The reason we keep steps small is because this means less impact and requires less braking, giving you better control of your stride. Keep steps fast and light, bobbing and weaving your body down the hill, using your arms for balance.'

Some other things to remember when you are running downhill include:

**Posture** – Tighten your core to stabilise your body and try to avoid leaning too far forwards or backwards. When you are new to downhill running there is a tendency to lean back to 'put the brakes on' and this can increase impact on your knees. Leaning forwards too much, although seemingly good for propulsion, can lead to a loss of control. Keri confirms this: 'A great position is to be landing directly over your feet, keeping your centre of gravity stable.'

**Foot placement** – Aim to land midfoot to minimise impact. Avoid heavy heel strikes, which can cause undue stress on your joints and lead to overstriding. Use your toes and feet to control your descent and stay agile, especially if you are on uneven terrain.

**Descend like a child** – Have you ever watched a child running downhill? Arms splayed out, running fast, joy on their faces. Well, I want you to remember that image when running downhill. I want you to use those arms for balance, too. Extending them out to your sides will help your body to naturally stabilise, especially on steeper or uneven terrain. Yes, you might feel silly at first but, I guarantee, you'll feel more stable and confident in your downhill running doing it.

> **RECAPTURE THE JOY**
>
> Keri: 'Often, women will say to me, "I haven't had that much fun in ages. I feel like a kid again!" We often forget to run with joy as adults; running downhill can help us recapture that feeling.'

**Practice makes perfect** – The more you practise running uphill and downhill, the more confident you will get. It will take time, so be patient with it, but know that consistency will breed confidence. There is fun to be had in hill training, so allow yourself the grace to play around, be childlike and know that – as the months and years pass – you will become a more efficient hill runner.

Hill running offers mounds of opportunity. For me, as a woman, learning to run uphill and downhill has meant I can run in places that I only ever saw in picture books. I have stood on top of local hills that, as a kid, I looked at and wondered, 'How do you get there?' I have climbed to mountain summits, as an adult, that I never ever thought were places for 'someone like me'.

So just remember . . . It's a hill: get over it.

CHAPTER 8

# Safety matters

Not feeling safe is a massive barrier to women using running as an activity to enhance their physical and mental well-being. For many women – maybe even you – it's the number one reason why they are reluctant to take it up.

I wish I could tell you that there is nothing to worry about, but we know that is not true. And – if I'm being honest with you – I know far too many women who have had negative experiences that have caused them to consider whether running is an appropriate way for them to spend their time.

> A 2024 survey by the University of Manchester showed that 82 per cent of female respondents said they worried about their personal safety while out running.

So many different aspects feed into feelings of anxiousness and fear around female running. Although we share many common concerns, the experience of running is different for each one of us due to the intersections that we inhabit, including race, disability, faith, body composition, mental health and more.

The top safety concerns for female runners are:

- Running at night
- Catcalling/verbal abuse
- Physical abuse
- Running alone

- Being followed
- Getting lost

The above is by no means a definitive list, and there will no doubt be other safety concerns that come into your mind.

No woman's experience is the same and some women will say that they have never felt a sense of fear when out running. And for them I am so happy, for they are the lucky ones. An Our Streets Now survey found that: 'over 70% of people had experienced sexual harassment while exercising or playing sports and 4 in 5 people make adjustments to their behaviours while exercising because of harassment or intimidation.'

I am a mother of three females. I will always fight for a society where every woman – no matter who they are – feels safe, supported and seen when they are moving their bodies in the outdoors. It's NOT OK – it will never be OK – for women to feel unsafe when doing something, an activity, that is promoted as *inclusive for all*.

Because, while other people – and by that I mean men – can just go out for a run with no thought for personal safety, our experiences as women can be very different.

So let me share my tips and advice to make you as safe as you possibly can be while on your running journey.

Shavaun is a female member of a UK-based running community.

### A LESSON IN MENTAL RESILIENCE AND WHAT NOT TO DO

Shavaun: 'It began when I lined up to collect my bib number. I handed over my ID only to witness a female volunteer do a double take when she saw my surname (I am of Black ethnicity). The awkward pause that followed was unmistakable, with her looking at me and then back to the document, as if trying to reconcile what she saw.

To have to experience this, at this event, while already feeling anxious due to being one of very few Black women on the start line, fed into feelings of isolation and doubt as to whether I should be there.

'But it didn't stop there because, just three miles into the race, the first blow came. As I passed them, a group of five male runners decided this was the perfect opportunity to make negative comments about my running. And then, blow two, another group of five male runners began reciting a version of a song from the musical *Oliver*, implying that I was not wearing or could afford standard running clothing. The song only appeared to get louder, emphasising certain words, such as "orphan", as they ran beside me and overtook me.

'Blow three – another two male participants running past me who intentionally slowed down to make derogatory comments. One came close to me, looked me up and down then said, "These professional runners!" – I assume commenting on my pace in comparison to theirs.

'And the final blow, being denied a fundamental human right – water! After crossing the finish line, I approached a female volunteer – I was exhausted mentally and physically – and asked for two cups of water. Her reluctance to give them to me was evident and she dared to challenge me in front of my family as if I was not a participant. Even after the race was over, I had to fight for my most basic needs.'

## Hello darkness, my old friend

As I'm writing this the clocks went back to Greenwich Mean Time (GMT), meaning that, for us UK-based runners, darkness descends before 4.30 p.m. So if we haven't had time to get our run done earlier, we must make the decision to run in the dark.

And running, especially if we run on our own, in the dark can be anxiety-inducing. How much or how little anxiety you will feel depends greatly on your lived experience and what you have seen or heard that has seeped into your consciousness about being a woman in the outdoors at night. I work in this space and am very conscious of local and national incidents that have involved female runners. I cannot guarantee, and no one can, that you will be 100 per cent safe but, if you do decide to run at night, the following measures will ensure that you have all of the mental and physical resources you need.

## Buddy up

Running solo is fine – and it will be a part of your running journey – but running with a friend or family member (preferably a human but a canine will also suffice) is better. You might not know anyone else who runs, or feel embarrassed to ask, but I guarantee you that there will be other women local to you who want company too.

Look online for local running groups that cater for new runners (for readers in England, the England Athletics RunTogether website is a resource to use. Just put in your postcode and hey presto, running groups galore!). I created my own female running community in 2016 and I encourage my members to communicate with each other about buddying up on runs in the evening.

Asking someone to run with you is a great way to not only keep you safe – because there's someone else there to help in case something happens *and* there's power in numbers – but it's also a great way to make new friends. I know it might feel scary – for fear of people saying no – but believe me when I say there *will* be a woman out there who feels the same way you do. They are looking for you!

A friend of mine, and someone I respect hugely, is Mel Bound. She is founder and CEO of This Woman Runs (TWR) – the largest social running network for women globally.

Mel founded TWR when her daughter was 18 months old. She had fallen out of love with running and injured her back, which led to major surgery and months of rehab. Struggling to adjust to life as a new mother, and without running, which was so central to her identity, Mel became completely inactive. She wondered how, if she was finding it hard as someone who had always previously been active, new mums who had never been active before were coping and making time to look after themselves. A post she put on Facebook led to 75 mums turning up to meet her for a run.

> **MEANINGFUL CONNECTION**
>
> Mel: 'I can still remember the euphoria of that first run. It was only for 5–10 minutes down the road but, for me, it became that light-bulb moment when I realised, "Oh wow. There are lots of us feeling like this!" It wasn't even about the running: it was about the moment of connection with women who feel just like you. I knew I had stumbled onto something really meaningful and that's how This Mum Runs – now named This Woman Runs – was born.'

## Light it up

If you are running at night then I really do advise that you run with a head or chest torch. You need to be able to see where you are going, and people need to be able to see you coming! There are perfectly good, value-for-money head torches available that throw out a decent amount of light, so do shop around. A head torch will sit on your forehead and is normally attached to a wide, stretchy, adjustable band that wraps around your head.

A chest torch normally has a couple of adjustable straps for your shoulders and chest. The light will usually sit at the front of your chest, underneath your breasts.

Weight, brightness, ease of use, cost, comfort and stability are all key factors when deciding which head torch to buy. You may hear people talking about 'lumens' – the brightness of the head torch – and, as a general rule you are looking for:

- General running (urban areas, parks, etc.) – a minimum of 300 lumens
- Technical running (trails, etc.) – 300–800 lumens

In terms of power, head torches normally run on AA, AAA or rechargeable batteries. But always remember to check the power *before* you go out on your run. I've lost track of the number of times I've got ready to go out running at night, switched on my head torch and been hit with a dead battery. It can be super annoying and, if you are looking for an excuse to bail on a run, then this happening can be it! I think that's why, for you as a beginner runner, I'd recommend a head or chest torch that takes AA or AAA batteries. They are quicker to replace, and you don't have to wait around for them to charge.

### Let's reflect

Running at night is about being visible. About selecting items of clothing that ensure motorists, cyclists and other road and track users can see you ahead of or behind them. There is a variety of reflective clothing on the market, which ranges in price. When I started running and knew that I would need to run at night, I purchased a cheap, pink running tabard that could be easily slid on over my jacket. The tabard featured a large reflective strip at the front and back. I remember that, to test it, I stood in the garden and had my husband shine a torch at me – just to check it worked.

Please, whatever you do, do not go out at night without some form of reflective kit on. I have seen too many people running in the dark in colours that, on dimly lit streets, make them impossible to see. You should also wear bright colours during the day if you are going to be running on roads where there are areas of deep shadow, since you will be very hard to spot if you are wearing black and drivers' eyes are adjusting to changing light levels as they go in and out of shade. Be safe, be seen!

## Running alone

I know many women who originally hated the idea of going out alone and now actively crave that me-time in their week. They yearn for those moments when they can leave it all behind and *just run,* time when they don't have to talk to anyone or be answerable to anyone. A run where they can zone out and focus on moving their bodies forwards in whatever way feels good to them.

I'm going to be honest with you: I have been known to cancel runs that were planned with friends because I just needed to be alone. To not have to worry about going too fast or slowing down for someone else.

And often to cry. Yes, running is my moving therapy, and sometimes I just need to stand on a trail and cry out loud without fear, judgement or questioning.

But when running alone there are some key things to remember to keep yourself safe.

## Have a fully charged mobile phone

Always ensure that you are carrying a *fully charged* mobile phone and that it is kept secure and easily accessible to you – or someone else, should they need it – via your pocket or a piece of kit such as a bum bag or waist belt. If you need to, you should always be able to contact someone if you are feeling anxious or need help. Also, make sure to include in case of emergency (ICE) details in your phone contacts list (listed as 'ICE – Name') so anyone who needs access to your emergency details can easily find them. Many phones have medical ID and SOS Emergency buttons that can be accessed if you are in need – please ensure these are kept updated. It's also important to point out that some sports watches (if you ever come to purchase one) have an 'emergency' setting that can be activated. The watch I wear has a fall detector that alerts someone if the watch experiences significant impact.

## Headphones

These days, wearing headphones is something that I advise against, whether running during the day or at night. It is really important for your safety to be aware of your environment. For example, there may be people who want to pass you (normally bike riders who don't seem to know how to use a bell!), dogs that approach you, traffic passing by close to you. Being conscious of what is going on around you – and within you – when running alone is so important. If you want to run with headphones to listen to your favourite podcast or music, then keep the volume low and only have one earbud in.

Over the years there has been a rise in different ranges of 'open ear' headphones. These products feature bone-conducting technology and convert sound into mechanical vibrations that are transmitted through the skin and temporal bone to the cochlea in the ear. They allow you to hear sound from the audio you have selected and to hear what is going on around you, too. These types of earphones are now my favourites because you can wear them in both ears and still hear what's going on around you.

## Location services

My husband can keep track of where I am (as can my children, unfortunately!) via an app that tracks me and is built into my phone. Now, I know that some people hate the idea of others knowing where they are at every minute of the day, but when it comes to personal safety for female runners, I do feel that we should make the most of the technology that is out there. Apps such as Find My Friends and similar allow hourly, daily or ongoing access for others to see your real-time location. Pick an app that works for you and give someone you trust access to track you on it.

## I'm off!

Always let someone know *when* you are going for a run, *your proposed route* and *when you estimate you will be back*. If you go out for a run that should take 40 minutes and you are not back in 90 minutes, then it is important that someone is aware of that. They need to be able to check you are OK. I have been out longer than intended many times – mostly on purpose – due to me taking more walk breaks than I had initially intended, or because I kept stopping to take a picture of a beautiful view or my sweaty face! But there have been a few times when my lateness back home has been due to something more serious, like going over on my ankle or not paying attention and falling over a tree root, meaning that my route took a lot longer than anticipated. Always share the above information with someone before you venture out.

## Don't lose yourself

Have you ever been lost? I have and it doesn't feel good at all. Whenever it happens to me, and these days it's normally when I am undertaking silly distances in running events, I always promise myself never to be in that situation again. When we are lost, our levels of panic start to rise and we can make irrational decisions based off fear, not facts. The rise in cortisol and adrenaline can trigger our fight-or-flight response, leading to bad decision-making.

I want you to run – if you are out at night especially – on routes that you know. I want you to focus on the process of running, not the fear of getting lost. I want the only thing that you think about to be the running session that you are in – not the fear of taking a wrong turn and ending up somewhere unfamiliar to you. Finding new and fun routes can come next. But, for this journey I really want you to remember – when it comes to routes – to KISS (keep it simple, stupid).

However, if by some chance you do get lost, just stop (right now, thank you very much). Physically stop! Look around and ask yourself, 'When was the last time I was in familiar territory?' Take a moment to breathe slowly in and out (to combat feelings of panic and bring down your heart rate) and then turn round and walk back the way you came. Keep on walking until you are back on the route you had originally planned and in a place you recognise. Don't run, walk. And, if by some chance you cannot find your way back – which, considering the distances that I am going to be asking you to run, is unlikely – then stop once again. It's time to call for help. It's time to relay some critical information to someone else.

## GPS location apps

There are a host of apps, some better known than others, that can give you easy-to-understand co-ordinates locating where you are. This means that friends, family and – if you need them – emergency services know where you are to the square metre and can find you. You do not need to know how to read a map to use these apps. With some apps all you need to do is open them up from your phone and press a button. You'll then be given a three-word reference that will tell people where you are. I – and many thousands of others – use a service called what3words, but there are others.

Please find an app that works for you and become familiar with it *before* you start running. I can't stress enough the importance of people being able to locate you.

# Variety is the spice of life

There are lots of different types of bad behaviour and abuse we might encounter when outdoors running, from verbal abuse in the form of catcalling and unwelcome comments on our bodies, to physical abuse such as unwanted touching, grabbing, groping or kicking (*see* Tasha's story on p. 117). And let's be clear: *all* physical abuse is abuse, no matter how insignificant it may seem to the abuser. And then there's psychological abuse, which can take the form of us feeling watched or followed.

Every single form of unwanted attention that we, as women, experience while out running has an impact on our experience. An impact on us wanting to continue.

To keep yourself safe, it's important that you ensure your runs are varied in terms of route choice and the time of day – or night – that you venture outdoors. Not only will this benefit your running – because variety really is the spice of life – but it also means you cannot so easily be located by strangers. Think about it: if you go out at the same time every Tuesday, Thursday and Sunday, on the same route, that makes it easy for others to find you.

Of course, you will have your favourite routes – we all do – those ones that are super easy to do and that you don't have to think about. But there are simple ways to change them up. For example, do them in reverse at a different time of day. But please do vary them, especially if running solo.

## Fitness tracking apps

Be mindful of locking your personal settings down You might want to consider turning off, or setting to private, your location settings if you use fitness tracking apps. Often the activity that you record is sent to an online platform, which, unless you have restricted your settings, can be viewed by the public. There are ways to hide your start and end point and, if you want to, you can even hide your complete route so that only you can see it. You can, and should, choose who gets access to your run data, but remember that the default setting is almost always public.

## Catcalling/verbal abuse

I have been running for years now and, although it has given me so much physically and emotionally, it can also still cause anxiety. My heart rate can still creep up if I run past large groups (men and teenagers being the worst). Why? Because of the inevitable stares, hushed whispers, giggles and often – if they are feeling brave – catcalls. It shouldn't be something we have to be wary of but being female runners, it is.

If on a particular day I feel confident, am in a safe space and want to challenge this behaviour, I will stop and ask *why* this person(s) feels the need to say that to me or the group of women I am running with. I will tell them how the catcalling is received by us. How it makes us *feel*. How, for many women who are trying to increase their physical and mental wellness via running, being on the receiving end of catcalling can create so much anxiety that it makes them stop.

If I'm feeling safe to, I ask them how they would feel if someone did what they have just done to their mother, sister or a female they love. The common response is often silence or a muttered apology. I like to think that they might think twice about their actions next time a female runner passes them.

Some other things you should consider are:

- Don't retaliate – Most of the time these people are looking for a reaction. Often the best approach is to ignore them as if they don't exist.
- Report it – If the comments you receive while running are of a racial, sexual, homophobic or faith-based nature then they should be reported to the police. If it is appropriate, and you are able to, take details of the company, organisation or even school that the abuser(s) are from.
- Vary your routes – As detailed above.

## Physical abuse

No woman should be physically abused full stop, never mind while out on a run. All forms of physical abuse – no matter how small – are abuse and should not be tolerated.

We should not have to tolerate it.

I remember a time that I had finished leading a run with my women's running group and was taking them through a stretching session. An elderly man walked behind me and slapped my bum, laughing as he did it. I remember being shocked that he was so blasé about laying his hands upon me and, when I challenged him, he insinuated that I 'couldn't take a joke'. That this man felt he had a right to put his hands on me signifies, in some small sense, what we as women deal with day in, day out. Behaviour that has been normalised for women the world over. Did I tell him that it was in fact *not a joke*. Yes. Did he feel ashamed? No, I don't think he did. I think he felt that I was overreacting.

A slap on the bum may seem low-level abuse, but it is not. From strangers laying hands upon us, to 'overfriendly' runners (often male) that we may know whose touch is *too* familiar, to being physically or sexually assaulted while out on the run – none of it is OK.

### KICKED ON MY WAY TO PARKRUN

Tasha Thompson, founder of Black Girls Do Run UK, has this story: 'On Christmas Day 2023 I was kicked by one of two drunk men on my way to Parkrun. It happened while I was standing at a pedestrian crossing. I could see that they were drunk and, using instinct, moved as far away from them as possible. But it made no difference. I was kicked and, to add insult to injury, he looked straight at me and laughed. I didn't say anything, as I could see that he had a bottle in his hand. I got to the Parkrun but didn't want to dampen anyone's spirits, so I kept it to myself.

'It took me four hours to get myself out of the door for the next run I did. I wore mainly black, thinking, "Maybe if I hadn't been wearing a bright colour that day [Christmas red] they wouldn't have noticed me, kicked me and laughed at me." Of course, this is nonsense, but it impacted my confidence, leaving me wondering, "What could I have done to prevent this happening to me?"

> 'I shared this with my running community and their support was invaluable and led to me reporting this incident. I would never have let this stop me running or take away my running joy but it really is tough for us women sometimes.'

## Report it

Tasha had the courage, and support, to report her experience to the police. But, in the survey by the University of Manchester, 95 per cent of women respondents said that they didn't report the abuse they'd encountered. Women gave a variety of reasons for not reporting an incident, including:

- The abuse of women in public is so normalised that their experiences are perceived as trivial.
- Incidents are often not judged as being criminal offences.
- They didn't want to waste police time.
- They had doubts about whether the police would be interested.

Abuse impacts us in so many ways, consciously and subconsciously. I want you to feel safe, to be prepared and to feel empowered to seek help if you need it, be that socially, professionally or legally.

If you feel the need, you can carry some products to ward off unwelcome advances:

- Farb gel spray
- Personal alarms

Many women run with a key in their hand, held between the fingers, but please note that in the UK it is illegal for any member of the public to carry a lethal or non-lethal self-defence weapon. This includes keys. It is also illegal for any member of the public to purchase, acquire or possess any item that discharges any form of gas, liquid or something else illegal. This includes pepper spray.

If you are abused, *please* tell someone. A friend, family member or stranger. Please do not carry the experience alone. You did not do anything to warrant being attacked. It is not your fault. I repeat: it is not your fault! My advice is to, with the support of a close confidante, report what has happened to the police. As women we may not know what other incidents have been reported, and you having the courage to report yours might be the trigger needed for resources to be allocated for further investigation. Your courage in reporting might stop another woman experiencing this abuse too. Your voice matters.

## Safety in numbers – the power of community

For many women, verbal and physical abuse comes because of the intersectionality that they inhabit as female runners. For some women, no amount of changing their routes, going out during the day or night, wearing reflective clothing, head torches or running in groups can stop them being targeted. Who are these women? These are Muslim women, women of colour, trans women, gay women, less able-bodied women, women experiencing invisible illnesses. All experience – or know someone who has experienced – physical and verbal abuse by virtue of being *who they are.*

I am a mixed-race woman of colour, racialised as Black, and due to the colour of my skin I almost lost my life while participating in an ultra-marathon (55K) in the Swiss Alps. Why? Because when I was walking along a narrow mountain path, a path that was still covered in snow even though it was July, I lost my footing and slipped off the path onto the side of the mountain. With every ounce of my strength I tried to grip onto snow (which was quickly melting in my hands) and rock, screaming for my life. Screaming for help. Every second, falling a little further. Not one of the white male runners who passed me helped me. My question, had I been able to ask it, to the runners who left me hanging there would have been, 'Had I presented as white – and looked more like your mother, sister or someone you cared about – would you have reached for me sooner?'

For months after, and still to this day, I feel a sense of anxiety about this happening again. Will my ethnicity impact how other people interact with me – or help me – while on a run?

And I know that I am not the only one. I know this because I am friends with women who due to their racial identity, due to wearing modesty clothing for religious or personal reasons, due to their body composition, have been targeted and have felt fear for their physical and mental safety while moving their body.

Often it is for reasons of safety, of being around other women who *get it*, that female-only running communities have been set up. Communities like This Woman Runs (TWR), or my own community, Stroud Mums on the Run. The communities my friends have set up – Black Girls Do Run UK and ASRA – were launched due to a need for women to feel safe, to feel seen and to run together as one.

I have felt so held – physically and mentally – when running in a community of women of differing intersectionalities who share elements of my lived experience. I know that they just get it. They understand it while we run together in the silent moments, in the reflective moments, in the 'Why does this feel so hard today, I can't do it' moments. They understand as mothers, as professional women trying to juggle, as women living with depression, as women of colour.

I am an advocate of finding your people and keeping them close. Believe me, there is a community out there for you, if you want one. Just have the courage to look for it.

## Not all men

I wish I didn't have to write a chapter like this. The last thing I want to do is put the fear of God into you. I know what fear does. I know how crippling it can be. But I hope that, by sharing advice on tools to use, kit to look at, must-dos and don'ts in this chapter, I have empowered you in some way.

Ultimately, the missing – and most important – piece in all of this is addressing the root cause of the problem: some men. It is society's responsibility to teach men *not* to assault women in the first place.

> An Adidas survey found that 92 per cent of 4,500 women in nine countries reported feeling concerned for their safety when they go out for a run.

I encourage women – and male allies – to speak up on issues of safety. Active bystanding is a way that we can support each other. It means taking action when we witness unacceptable, harmful or inappropriate behaviour. It means speaking up, intervening and offering support to prevent or stop harm. It means not ignoring it.

Ultimately, putting the responsibility of 'safety' on us women is a barrier to the change that we need to see. I know that, and that's why, as someone who fights for equity and equality, writing this chapter feels strange because, in a sense, it shifts the focus away from the real problem: the actions of some men.

The irony of that is not lost on me.

All I can hope is that, by sharing the tools and strategies I have, that you feel safer. That you feel supported. And that you can be the inspiration that other female runners need to see to feel that they too can start running.

## CHAPTER 9

# Don't stop, period!

I started my period at 11 years old. I remember the day I looked down and saw the spots of fresh red blood, and with it, the abject fear that consumed me. The cause of this fear was the fact that I was becoming a woman – well, that's what I remember the sex education teacher at school telling me. And this, my first period, was a sign that the change was happening. That my body was mature enough to grow a baby! I hated that feeling. Because I wasn't ready to be a woman or have a baby and I didn't want my bloody period.

Some of you older women reading this will remember the school 'talk' about the birds and bees. Of a video being played that showed a drawing of a vagina and a uterus. A voiceover that told us, in simple terms, what happens during a 28-day cycle. Was anyone else sent home with a small 'feminine' pack that included a tampon, a sanitary towel and a small instruction booklet on how to use them both?

The salient points back then – and today – were that periods were the sign of a healthy female body doing what it needed to prepare itself to do what it has done for thousands of years: to produce children. That was the only message that I remember.

I don't remember being told that periods can be so painful they can make you sick. That they can be so light as to be barely there or so heavy you might feel you are dying. That, due to the hormones involved, they can make you overly emotional, highly anxious and depressed. That they can make you feel like you want to eat the whole cake aisle at the local supermarket.

I don't remember being told that every single one of us will experience our menstrual cycle in different ways or how important periods are to a women's biological and psychological well-being.

Or how not having a period – unless you have an underlying health condition, are using contraception that means you don't have periods, or are pregnant – meant that something was seriously off kilter.

But there are a few things that I do remember, the first being that, when it came to participating in PE at school, I and my girlfriends could get a free pass out of the class if we had our period. This was a pass that many of us used because the humiliation of doing PE with a big, bulky sanitary pad, or leaking through our gym shorts, would mean social suicide.

I remember my mum giving me a hot water bottle when I had period pains and telling me to lie down, close the curtains and rest. How the best place for me was 'in bed' until it passed.

And I can't help but feel that this generational fear around women and periods – and exercising during the menstruation part of your cycle especially – is still with us today. I see it. I see women in the process of learning to run who are not well informed about how their menstrual cycle can work with, not against, them; who stay indoors for fear of the pain, of bleeding out, of being too fatigued to do it. Because they believe through misinformation that running will cause more harm than good.

That's not true.

> In 2022, the UK charity Women in Sport (WIS) surveyed 4,000 teenage girls and found that 78 per cent of them said they avoid sport when they have their period.

## Busting the period myth

The WIS survey found that 59 per cent of teenage girls who used to be sporty like sport but that they 'are being failed due to early years stereotyping, inadequate opportunities, and a complete dearth of knowledge about managing female puberty.'

Teenage girls like you – because I know there will be teenage girls reading this book, too – and female adults have always liked being active. But there are fears that need to be addressed. The most common things that stop people exercising during their period are:

- Pain and cramps
- Fatigue and low energy
- Bloating and discomfort
- Managing flow and leaks
- Feeling self-conscious

Renee McGregor is a leading sports dietitian specialising in RED-S (relative energy deficiency in sport), the female athlete, hormonal health and athlete performance. She is also my friend and my go-to on all things related to the menstrual cycle.

She says: 'I believe the reticence that there can be when it comes to women wanting to engage in running when they have their periods stems from negative generational discourse around menstruation. We were told by our mothers, and them by their mothers, that we "don't talk about periods". That we "don't do much when on our period". Almost as if our period makes us a pariah. A person that others should not go near. That narrative, to this day, continues to filter down into how we, as females, move our bodies during our menstrual cycle.'

## Textbook!

One thing that it is key to remember is that you are not textbook. There is no such thing when it comes to the female cycle. How you experience your menstrual cycle is unique to you. It's so important that – to enjoy the process of learning to run – you start to get to know the signs and symptoms that you experience during each phase of your cycle. Because to be forewarned is to be forearmed.

From a biological point of view, you will normally experience four key phases of your cycle and, for you as a woman who wants to learn to run, it's really important to understand not only what these are, but also how these phases will impact on your thoughts, feelings and biological responses to running. Understanding how fluctuating hormone levels might affect you will help you also understand what types of running might work better for you at different times of the month.

Below is a summary of each phase of the menstrual cycle and a guide to approximate days of your cycle when you might start to see changes occur. Please remember that a woman's menstrual cycle can last between 21 and 35 days (the average is 28). And, for some teenage girls, cycles can be as short at 20 days or as long as 45 days. I'll say it again: the only normal when it comes to a menstrual cycle is what's normal for you.

## The menstrual cycle

| Day | Phase | What's going on? |
| --- | --- | --- |
| 1–5 | Menstrual – you've started bleeding | Your hormone levels (oestrogen and progesterone) are at their lowest. You might experience pain and cramps, fatigue and heavy bleeding (especially at the start of your period). |
| 6–13 | Follicular – just after your period | Your oestrogen level is beginning to rise but your progesterone level remains low. Your energy level starts to increase – yay! |
| 14 | Ovulatory – mid-cycle | Your oestrogen is at its peak and there's a surge of luteinising hormone (LH), which leads to ovulation. At this stage you may feel like superwoman – your energy and strength are often at their highest at this time. |
| 15–28 | Luteal – the time before you get your period | Your progesterone level rises and your oestrogen level fluctuates. You may feel more sluggish and experience bloating, cravings or mood swings as your body prepares for menstruation. |

## Keep track

Back in the day, I kept track of one thing to do with my period – the day it came. I only did this because there was no way I wanted to be at school or work and bleed onto my clothes. I didn't understand the importance of logging other symptoms – and didn't know enough to care, either.

Nowadays, there are a host of apps that can be used to log your menstrual cycle and symptoms associated with it. My advice is to start doing it, today. Starting to understand your body will not just help you on this running journey, but in life. Find a way to log that works for you. I'm old-school: I like writing things down in a notebook. I give myself five minutes at the beginning or end of the day. I sit in silence and tune in. It's during that time that I record how I feel physically, mentally and, if I have run that day, what that felt like.

By starting to keep track of how you feel during different phases of your cycle, you will see patterns emerge, which will empower your running and help, ultimately, with adherence and goal-setting.

## Dealing with symptoms

> **HORMONAL FATIGUE**
>
> 'I get so tired. My heart rate always rises higher not only while running but for the period after as well. I feel unable to go faster or run longer and it takes me longer to recover from a run. Prescription iron and a high-iron diet have helped me.'

During your menstrual cycle, due to fluctuating hormone levels, there will be some types of running that you will feel better doing than others. There will be times you feel like superwoman and want to run faster or do an additional run up a hill. There will be times when even running for a minute feels like hard graft. It's helpful to remember that your menstrual cycle massively influences how you feel and what you can do.

Here's an idea of what types of running might work better during the phases of your menstrual cycle.

## Menstrual – you start to bleed

**Likely symptoms:** Pain and cramps. Fatigue. Light to heavy bleeding.

**Try:** Perform a gentle warm-up incorporating a five-minute walk followed by some stretches that target the lower abdomen – stretches like a cobra pose, a supine stretch, or a cat cow (which will stretch your lower abdominals as well as your lower back). Some stretches for the lower back include a child's pose and a supine knee-to-chest stretch, among others. Examples of these stretches can be easily found online.

**Running:** This is a time for gentle aerobic run/walking. We're not interested in personal bests or faster running on these days. We want to get you out for non-strenuous movement that stimulates the release of inflammation-reducing endorphins.

## Follicular – just after your period

**Likely symptoms:** You'll feel like you're coming out of your slump, with energy levels starting to increase. Your recovery time, both during and post run, will also be faster.

**Try:** This is a great time for you to play around with seeing what you can do. The energy boost you are experiencing might make you feel more capable of trying running sessions that are of a higher intensity.

**Running:** This phase is a great time to incorporate speedier sessions, interval training or slightly longer periods of faster running. It's a time for challenging yourself and ensuring appropriate fuelling around your runs. Think about your carbohydrate intake before and your carbohydrate and protein mix immediately after (*see* p. 201).

## Ovulatory – mid-cycle

**Likely symptoms:** You're going to be feeling amazing – on top of the world. Your energy and strength are at their highest. However, it's important to remember that the rise in oestrogen can increase your joint laxity, which might make you more prone to injuries like strains or sprains. So be careful out there, superwoman!

**Try:** Ensure you prepare for your running sessions by warming up adequately and following the mobility drills described in chapter 7 and the Miles and Smiles chapter on page 212. Ensure your body is ready for what you will be feeling emboldened to ask it to do.

**Running:** It might be during this phase of your cycle that you test yourself on a section of a route or a hill that has been a 'goal' during your running journey. Or it might be during this phase of your cycle that you decide to complete your 'goal' 5K run, which you'll do at the end of the 10-week programme.

## Luteal – the time before you get your period

**Symptoms:** I'm sorry but you're going to start to feel sluggish again. You may experience bloating, cravings (often sugar) and mood swings as your body prepares for menstruation. Your breathing might also feel more laboured, and you may sweat more.

**Try:** If running feels like one step too far on a particular day then try cross-training – yoga, swimming, cycling or strength and conditioning (see chapter 11 for some ideas). Pick something that feels manageable for how your body and mind feel on a particular day.

**Running:** Everything is going to feel more challenging due to an increased perceived rate of exertion combined with a decreased feeling of wanting to run. During the luteal phase, as hormones are fluctuating, your energy requirements will go up due to a higher core temperature, which is why we crave food. Additionally, progesterone can cause fluctuations in your blood sugar, so ensuring regular intake of carbohydrate and protein snacks can help prevent this. Your body will probably be more dependent on carbohydrates during this phase. Prioritise recovery and really listen to what your body is telling you. If you need to rest, then do that. Do not push through a training run if you feel fatigued.

> **LISTEN TO YOUR BODY**
>
> 'The week before my period it is hard to do anything, let alone run. We're supposed to take it easy and eat. That's what I do!'

# Why running during your menstrual cycle matters

Remember those top five fears that women had when running during their menstrual cycle? Well, far from running making them worse, it can help to lessen them! I'm not joking. Let me tell you more.

## Pain and cramps

If you experience period pain and cramps then you'll know how debilitating they can be. I am lucky in the sense that I have never suffered too badly, but I know women who do and, sister, if you are one of them, my heart goes out to you. I know that when experiencing period pain and cramps the last thing you might want to do is go out for a run but, believe me when I say, it can help to lessen pain. Why? There are a few reasons:

- Running will improve the circulation of your blood, which will help to reduce pain and cramps. Better blood flow will flush out pesky prostaglandins – the hormone-like chemical that is responsible for cramps. Be gone!

- Running will trigger the release of endorphins, which are your body's natural painkillers. They'll reduce the perception of pain while increasing your feel-good factor.
- Running will make you relax. The rhythmic movement of running can help to relax your uterine muscles, which in turn will reduce the intensity of cramps. If you suffer from back pain, too – as many women do – running can also alleviate tension there.

## Fatigue and low energy

As you now know, there are going to be specific times during your cycle when you are going to feel much more fatigued. You'll feel like you can't be arsed to even lift your hand to your mouth to get that last bit of cake in, never mind go out and run! Remember, this is normal! During these phases – mostly the menstrual and luteal phases – your body is working super hard in the background doing its natural thing. So, while it does that, use running to give yourself a natural boost.

- Running will deliver more oxygen and nutrients to your muscles and brain, which, in turn, will make you feel more awake and energised.
- Running will give you that runner's high! Those endorphins will come into play once again.
- Running will help to regulate stress hormones such as cortisol and adrenaline. It's those high levels of cortisol that can lead to feelings of exhaustion, so reduce them and get out on a gentle run.
- Running will help improve the quality of your sleep, meaning you'll fall asleep faster and deeper. And better sleep = more energy.

## Bloating and discomfort

Sometimes my bloating can be so bad that I look as though I'm six months' pregnant. My tummy feels hard and even contemplating getting into a pair of elasticated shorts or leggings feels impossible. But . . .

- Running – due to its circulation-increasing benefits – will help your body to eliminate excess fluids that contribute to bloating. That sense of tightness in the abdominal area will feel reduced.
- Running gets you moving – literally! – and when I say 'moving' in this context, I mean your digestive tract. I tend to suffer from not being as regular as I would like. Running is the only thing that can often 'get things moving', aiding the passage of gas and food from inside me to outside me. It helps me poo – there, I said it. If I am feeling bloated, running is my go-to release valve. Believe me, even a 10-minute run is enough to help things shift!
- Running will help eliminate water and salt – due to sweating – which will help reduce puffiness and that bloated feeling caused by water retention. But also remember, dehydration can worsen bloating, so be sure you drink water before and after you go out.

## Managing flow and leaks

> **MANAGE YOUR PERIODS**
>
> 'My period has affected my running due to pain and concerns about bleeding in public. I take daily iron supplements and use birth control in order to manage my periods so that I can run consistently.'

Do you know what is the number one thing that stops women from running during the luteal and menstruation phase of their cycle? The fear of their own blood. The fear of running along and blood – unbeknown (or known) to them – seeping through their pants, shorts or leggings for all to see. The thought of blood running down their leg – oh, the shame of it! The humiliation of this happening is so frightening that it stops women dead in their tracks. It stops women from benefitting from all the positives that running during these stages can give them.

Have I leaked while on my period? Yes, I have. Did it happen during the first few days of the menstrual phase when I had a heavier flow? Yes, it did. Would you, as a passer-by, have known it was happening? Absolutely not. Why? Because I was prepared for it. Because I knew, from tracking my cycle, that my period was either due to come or – because I could physically see it before I started to run – was there. And because I knew this, I was prepared to deal with it.

I am sick and tired of feeling shame when it comes to something natural happening to me. I have a period. So what? I bleed! So what? So, how do you handle it? Here are some tips:

- If you are on your period, choose a high-absorbency tampon, sanitary towel (my tip is to go for one with wings, as the movement of running can cause them to move around), a menstrual cup (a small, soft silicone cup that can be inserted into the vagina to collect blood) or period-proof underwear. I love the invention of period-proof underwear because, for me, wearing a pair of these gives me added security that, even if I am wearing a super-absorbent tampon and do leak, the underwear will soak it up. And you can get different products for different flow days. When I've finished my run, I simply take them off and throw them in the washing machine (check the label – some need a cold wash, and no fabric conditioner; you might also want to rinse them in cold water first). I also carry a spare product like a tampon or a sanitary pad, just in case.
- This feels like a no-brainer but sometimes the best tips are: I advise that you wear black or dark-coloured shorts or leggings to hide potential leaks. I mostly run in dark bottom layers, mainly because I prefer them, but also because if I leak, fall on my bum or have another accident, it doesn't show as much!
- Wear snug, but not tight, running clothes on those days you are feeling heavier or bloated. You want to pick clothes that offer you

comfort and support but also allow your body to breathe. Overly tight clothes that feel too restrictive can add to your overall feelings of discomfort.

- Run on routes that you know. During this phase you might like to pick a route that takes you past a public toilet or supermarket. Sometimes just knowing that, if needs be, there is somewhere to check yourself or change a tampon can give you the confidence to get out.

## Feeling self-conscious

It's easy to feel self-conscious, but if you follow the advice above, hopefully you will feel better. You should also know that most people have no idea that you're on your period. No matter what you think, other people passing you are more focused on their own activities than yours.

By using running as a means of managing symptoms associated with your menstrual cycle you are fostering an empowering way to care for yourself. Go you!

---

**BANISH THE SHAME**

'I do get very heavy periods and, during runs, have bled through multiple pads. I have found that using period underwear does help but – also – I am working through my embarrassment. Periods are natural. They are part of life and, as a woman, of creating life. They are nothing to be ashamed about, ever.'

---

# Heart rate training and the menstrual cycle

In chapter 5 I spent a lot of time talking about how to train using rate of perceived effort. I talked about how that perceived effort is based on truly understanding how you feel on any given day when it comes to energy availability for your running sessions. During your menstrual cycle, due to fluctuating hormone levels and the demands placed on your body, your heart rate will of course fluctuate.

When it comes to running, it's that correlation between heart rate and perceived effort that matters to me, and I want it to matter to you. Keeping an eye on your resting heart rate (RHR) – and heart rate variance overall – is a great way to really tune into what's happening. In general:

**During your period (menstrual):** RHR may be lower than your norm.

**After your period (follicular):** RHR is at your normal range and may start to increase.

**Mid-cycle (ovulation):** RHR will peak.

**Just before your period (luteal):** RHR might be higher.

---

### WHAT IS MY RHR?

Your resting heart rate is your heart rate when you are completely at rest, such as first thing in the morning before you get out of bed. To take it, find your pulse on your neck or wrist and count the number of beats in 30 seconds and then times that by two. If you have a smart watch that monitors heart rate, you can obviously use that, too.

---

## Heart rate variance (HRV)

This refers to the variance in the time intervals between consecutive heartbeats. It is a key indicator of the balance between the sympathetic (fight-or-flight) and parasympathetic (rest-and-digest) branches of your automatic nervous system. Your HRV is influenced by various internal and external factors.

Over the past five years I have kept an eye on my heart rate variance as an indicator of what might be happening to me that I can't 'see' – or don't want to! And it was Renee McGregor who alerted me to the importance of using HRV as a way to understand the times when my body might be working hard without me being aware of it. Whether that was when I was in a specific phase of my cycle, under emotional stress, fighting illness or – in my case – lacking iron.

If you want to measure HRV, the easiest – and most cost-efficient – way to do this is to use a smartphone camera paired with a HRV app (these apps can be found by simply searching for HRV wherever you download your apps). To measure your HRV you simply place your finger on the phone's camera and follow the app's instructions for measurement.

Renee explains why this is important: 'I encourage all of the women I meet to be aware of their heart rate variance. As women, we deal with stressors all the time, in all areas of our lives. We ask ourselves, "Why am I so tired? Why am I feeling groggy and coming down with colds and coughs a lot?" Keeping track of your HRV will give you clues as to the reasons why. Often, even when we think we are at rest, our body is still working really hard. And people don't realise that your body can be working hard without you doing anything. Especially during specific phases of our menstrual cycle.'

We are not machines. Our bodies can, and do, give us signals as to what they need. But we must be willing to listen, and that is why I advocate the running on feel method I described in chapter 5. This allows us to better tune into what is happening within our bodies and, along with keeping an eye on other factors, such as heart rate variance, can make this running journey – even when running on our period – dare I say it, a joyful experience!

# A helping hand

There are tons of over-the-counter medications and herbal remedies that you can take to alleviate menstrual symptoms, especially pain and cramps. You may decide, as many of us have, that popping a couple of paracetamol before a run will help you feel more confident to tackle to run. If so, do that. I'm not judging you. However, something else that you may want to try is starflower oil.

Renee advocates for its use, too: 'There is good, robust evidence to show that if you have heavy periods or experience mood swings and/or symptoms of fatigue, using starflower oil can be helpful. The reason being that it includes an essential fatty acid called gamma-linolenic acid (GLA).'

Renee advises that when buying starflower oil, you ensure it contains a high percentage of GLA: 'Make sure to compare different products and go for the one that has the higher percentage. Many companies that produce starflower oil aren't good at promoting GLA levels, but it is *the* ingredient that will support menstrual symptoms, so do your research.'

In chapter 12 I talk to Renee about food, drink and other supplements that will give our bodies the fuel they need to run joyfully. However, when it comes to fuelling to support you during your menstrual cycle, she advises that you aim to incorporate those foods that will help reduce inflammation. Examples are foods that are high in essential fatty acids, such as seeds, nuts and avocados. It's also super important to stay on top of your energy requirements. As women, we tend to fight our bodies when they send us signals that they are hungry, that they need calories. We'll drink a litre of water to quell hunger pangs rather than eat something. This is not going to help your body.

> Research shows that a woman's basal metabolic rate – the amount of energy (calories) your body requires to perform basic life-sustaining functions while at rest – increases by approximately 200 calories a day just before your period (luteal phase), so eat the darned carbohydrate. You need it!

Renee explains: 'The reason we as women crave sugar during different stages of our cycle, especially the luteal phase, is because our body needs that additional energy for vital processes to take place. Our body is working hard. It needs food. It needs calories. Part of the reason you are probably feeling hungry is because you have not ingested enough carbohydrate during the day. As women we must get into the habit of listening to our bodies and make informed choices based on what we know will not only fuel us but will also help to alleviate symptoms.'

## Why not getting your period is a red flag

As much as periods can be annoying, and can cause us discomfort both mentally and physically, they are a barometer for health. Having a period tells us that we are getting the balance right across the board. That balance being food, exercise and rest. A regular period tells us that we are functioning efficiently.

If you don't have a period – and do not have an underlying health condition, are not pregnant and are not taking a contraceptive such as a hormonal coil, which might mean you just don't get periods – then one of those areas might be out of kilter. And please know that the consequences of not having a period are serious.

According to Renee: 'You might think that it's great not to have a period, not to have to worry about it, but you'd be wrong. If you do not have a period, then that means you are not producing enough oestrogen, testosterone or growth hormone. Oestrogen is super important for bone health, and, in my work, I am seeing an increase in women who are having issues with their bone health, which present as fractures and breaks. These women may not have had a regular period for months and have not sought help because they deemed this as normal or something that would "right itself eventually". Or maybe they saw not having a period as "one less thing to worry about". Not having a period – if you are a woman who has no underlying health issue, nor is pregnant [or on contraception that affect the menstrual cycle] – is serious. Please seek expert help.'

I hope that in this chapter I have explained how you can still, and really should, continue to run when you are not only in the menstrual (bleeding) phase of your cycle, but throughout. I truly believe that taking time to understand your cycle and how it can supercharge your running can make you a stronger, more resilient runner. Tune in, in order to get out.

CHAPTER 10

# Menopause matters

I remember the first time I knew something was not quite right. That something, biologically, was shifting. That there was 'a change'.

And it scared the living daylights out of me.

Because I thought I might be dying.

It was 2016 and I was sitting in a coffee shop with my friend, Sarah. The day was just like any other, nothing remarkable – we were talking about life and the stresses of it. I remember moving my seat forwards to stand up and, as I did, I felt a massive gush of *something* escape from my vagina.

How can I describe that feeling? Well, you know when you go to turn on a tap too fast and the water comes gushing out in a powerful cascade. It was like that, but the tap was me and the *something* – upon looking down – was blood.

The surprise of it happening had me sitting back down, quickly. Because there was blood on the coffee shop floor. And I felt a wave of shame, embarrassment and fear.

I must caveat this experience by saying that I have never, when menstruating, had heavy periods. The only time in my life that I had experienced blood loss like I saw that day was during and immediately after giving birth to my four children. And I knew that I was not pregnant that day in the cafe.

So, what the hell was going on?

I wasn't prepared. I had no sanitary towels or tampons. I could see that the blood had seeped through my leggings for all to see if I let them. In that moment, I didn't know what to do. It reminded me of the day I had my first period, at school, as an 11-year-old.

But, at 38, I felt abject fear. Because this was not my normal.

I whispered what had happened to my friend, and she helped me clean up and escape that shop with what little dignity I felt I had left. She gave me a coat to wear around my waist and we got the hell out of there.

I had just experienced my first episode of 'flooding'.

It happened intermittently for months. Sometimes around the time of my period, often not. And every time it happened I became more fearful. Because, combined with symptoms of fatigue and a lack of energy and motivation for life in general, I thought I might be seriously ill. So, after months of dealing with it alone – and with a massive running challenge on the horizon – I made an appointment with my doctor.

## Flooding

I had never heard the term flooding before my doctor mentioned it to me as a symptom of perimenopause. And not only had I never heard this term for excessive bleeding, but I didn't think that – at 38 – I could be classified as perimenopausal. I was too young, surely? I thought that only women in their late 40s and 50s went through what my granny used to refer to as 'the change'.

But the symptoms that I was showing – flooding, fatigue and a lack of motivation for running (something that had become a lifeline to me) all pointed to that fact that I – at 38 – was in perimenopause.

> ### WHAT IS PERIMENOPAUSE?
>
> Perimenopause is the transitional phase leading up to menopause. It marks the time when our bodies begin to produce less oestrogen and other hormones in preparation for the end of the menstrual cycle. This phase can last for anything from a few months to over a decade, with the average duration being about five to seven years (with some women reporting longer than that). Perimenopause can begin from your mid-30s (or occasionally much younger) or as late as your 50s. When it starts depends on your genetics, lifestyle and overall health.

The thing I learned back then is there is no blood test that can tell you that you are in this phase. The only signs are the symptoms. And flooding is just one of very many. Here are some of the others:

- Hair loss
- Irritability
- Mood swings
- Hot flushes
- Anxiety and depression
- Brittle nails
- Allergies
- Dry, itchy skin
- Loss of libido

The fact that I was losing so much blood didn't help the intense fatigue I was feeling and – after a routine blood test – I was also diagnosed as anaemic. I was sent away with an information leaflet about perimenopause and hormone replacement therapy (HRT), a prescription for ferrous sulphate and an appointment to have a Mirena coil fitted (my doctor told me it would help lessen the bleeding).

But there was something else on my mind. How would being in perimenopause and, after that, menopause, affect my running? Would it make it harder? Did I need to train differently? Would I be more susceptible to specific niggles or injuries? Would the food and drink I had been using work the same way?

I had so many questions. And to me they were important questions that, at the time, I couldn't get answers to because the menopause advocacy movement that we see these days was not as prolific.

Those topics that are hidden away, that are not discussed for fear of us being stereotyped, passed over or 'put out to pasture', get stronger and scarier. I do not want a biological barrier to affect you learning to love running. Whether we like it or not, we will all go through these phases, either naturally or surgically.

You are not alone. I am here to tell you that, yes, you can still run. I am here to share what advice has worked for me and other women when it comes to starting and continuing to run in these stages. And, for the science and expert bit, I have enlisted the help of a menopause specialist to make you feel empowered as you go through these phases as a female runner.

> **PERIMENOPAUSE TO MENOPAUSE**
>
> You are officially in menopause a year after your last period. So, if you don't have a period and then get one six months later, you must start counting again from the date of that last period.

## No such thing as normal

When it comes to perimenopause and menopause it's important for you to remember that there is no such thing as normal. There is no one-size-fits-all. How a friend, family member or another female runner experiences them will be different. In terms of understanding your changing cycle and the symptoms associated with it, one thing that is advised is to start – if you don't already – to keep a diary. Note down information about when you menstruate and all the symptoms you experience so that you start to get a better grasp on what is happening and when. This means that, if you need to, you can refer back to it to track changes.

Menopause specialist Dr Cath Munro, who is a member of the British Menopause Society alongside being a general practitioner, hosts workshops that focus on perimenopause and menopause for female runners.

Cath says: 'I always say track your periods and track your symptoms. Be aware of what's going on because there's a lot that can change. You might have had PMS-type symptoms that, either suddenly or gradually, seem to be worsening. Some months might feel awful and others not too bad. If symptoms aren't bothering you and you think, "You know what, it's OK, I can deal with these", then that is great. You only need to address your symptoms if they are impacting on your life or are distressing and causing you anxiety.'

Here are some of the symptoms that female runners report they experience:

- Joint pain
- Increased recovery time
- Tendonitis issues
- Physical fatigue
- Mental fatigue
- Weight gain
- Hot flushes/running 'hot'

## Should I stop running?

Ultimately, whether you choose to go out for a run or not is a decision that only you can make but, from a medical perspective, no, you shouldn't stop running. Evidence shows that going out for a run – or doing any form of cardiovascular exercise – can help reduce your symptoms rather than making them worse.

## Joint pain

Joint pain and stiffness during perimenopause and menopause are common symptoms felt by all women, not just runners. These symptoms result from fluctuating hormone changes. The decline of oestrogen, which plays a significant role in maintaining joint and bone health, can trigger physiological symptoms that affect the joints. We'll talk more about the importance of strength training as a means of supporting joints, bones and tendons in the next chapter.

Cath has this to say: 'A big part of my job lies in reassuring women who might be experiencing joint pain, as an example, that they are not going to hurt themselves by running with these hormone-related aches and pains. By all means, if the joint pain is increasing your anxiety, which impacts on the joy you might feel when running, then go and get checked out. But I have seen that, and the evidence shows, exercise goes a long way in helping to reduce this symptom. Plus running in particular helps with other things like bone health, balance and mental well-being, too. There's really nothing to lose by trying it.'

> **WORK WITH YOUR BODY**
>
> 'Although I am not in perimenopause yet, I think I am close to it. I've experienced joint pain, especially in my knees and ankles, which has impacted my running. When that happens, I make sure to take it easy and focus on other forms of training, including strength training, spinning and yoga. This allows time for symptoms to ease. It's so important that I listen to my body and give it the rest it needs so I can resume running when I am ready.'

Look, I know how it feels. I have been there – I am there! There are days when I wake up with a run on the plan and it is the *last thing* I want to do. My back hurts for no identifiable reason, I am tired even though I have had my required eight hours of sleep, I feel bloated, yadda, yadda, yadda. *Everything* in my being tells me that I should roll over, stay in bed and weep about the unfairness of it all – because, you know, I'm overly emotional as well!

But I know that staying where I am and not even *trying* to run will make me feel much worse in the long term. I know that running will probably help to lessen the symptoms that I feel, even if I only run for 10 minutes.

And I know it can help you, too. It's never too late.

> **MY 5K AND ME**
>
> 'My mum enrolled me on a C25K course and gave it to me as a Christmas present. I had no idea what to expect but, as Mum had paid for it, I had to try. The coach, and women who were in the same

> boat, were so encouraging and – although I found out during the course that I had some health complications – I ran on "feel" and using a run/walk strategy, kept moving. Completing my first 5K, after 10 weeks, made me feel so proud of myself and make a connection with the women who have since become good friends.'

# Fatigue

For me, and I know for many other women, the increased feelings of fatigue that I have experienced during perimenopause has, at times, been really worrying. I'll admit that my increased levels of physical and mental fatigue – symptoms I will address separately below – have had me visiting the GP due to increased anxiety around a sense that 'this cannot be normal, something is really wrong'.

Tests have showed that I am not dying of an invisible illness. Fatigue is a symptom of perimenopause and one that I – and you – must find effective ways to deal with.

> 'My lord, the fatigue. How does it affect my running? Well, some days it feels like my legs are made of concrete. It looks like me not picking my knees up high enough, scuffing my feet during a run and, at times, tripping and falling. This leads to my confidence being knocked and has me asking, "Is this really a good thing for me to be doing?" It looks like my running pace slowing down, not being able to hit the speed that I once did. It feels like I am running on empty, that I do not have enough energy to complete sometimes even the shortest run. And guess what? All these symptoms can change daily, weekly or monthly.'

Mental fatigue can lead to symptoms such as increasing levels of irritability, anxiety, episodes of depression and just needing to stop life and take a minute. It can also lead to brain fog and forgetfulness.

My own experience? Some days you'll find me in my kitchen, sitting down, trainers on but not having a clue where I am going to go on a run. Not feeling as if I have the mental capacity to plan a route. Wanting a magical menopause fairy to appear and tell me where to go and what to do because I'm too mentally tired to even want to plan the run, never mind do it. But just getting out for 10 minutes can be a mood booster and can lift me out of those feelings of sadness and brain fog and literally clear my head. On these days the run is about the mood-boosting benefit of a short run; the physical benefit comes second.

And I *know* the power of running, I know how it can help alleviate these symptoms of fatigue. I've seen it in others and experienced it. But I also know that if I feel this way then there must be countless women out there going through this phase who feel that they can't – or shouldn't – even try.

But you should try because cardiovascular exercise – in our case, running – can minimise these symptoms. Here are some strategies that I employ that help me get through days when the fatigue feels overwhelming:

## You can do anything for 10 minutes

When even the thought of a run is too mentally exhausting, I remind myself that I can do *anything for 10 minutes*. I give myself express permission that, if I want to turn around and come back after this time, I absolutely can. That, even by completing 10 minutes, I have beaten everyone else on the sofa. I choose however I want to run during those 10 minutes, whether that is a run/walk, a shuffle or a jog. Talking to myself in this way often leads to me not just getting out but being out for longer than 10 minutes because once you're out, you might as well stay out.

## Mindful movement

Studies show that practising mindfulness and meditation can have an impact on feelings of fatigue. In chapter 5 we learned about running on feel. About being truly present in your body and mind during a run. About focusing on your body, your breath, your mind. Practising this way of mindful running has allowed me to better understand what might be contributing to feelings of fatigue. To give me headspace to think about what areas of my life might feel overwhelming and how I might be able to address that. And sometimes the only way I feel I can address feelings of fatigue is to . . .

## . . . Take a 'nanna nap'

I am a grandmother, so I am allowed to use this term! I love nanna naps – often referred to as 'disco naps' or siestas. Never underestimate the power of sleep for mental and physical health, and recovery from running. When the fatigue feels too much, I intentionally create time for a nap. That nap can take place during a lunch break or before or after a run. And the science backs this recovery protocol. Thirty minutes, for me, is the perfect length.

> **SLEEP CYCLES**
>
> Our sleep cycles are 30 minutes in length so, if you are going for a reinvigorating nap, decide how long your nap cycle will be and base it on 30-minute phases (30, 60 or 90 minutes). Any shorter or longer might leave you feeling groggy.

## Run with a friend

You know what can often get me out when I am feeling like I can't be bothered? Arranging to run with a friend! If I am feeling unmotivated and know I have a run coming up, I will reach out to a friend to see if they want to accompany me. Planning to run with someone else, at a certain time, can be just the trigger you need to go out. It's about accountability and connection to someone else who may feel the same way. I have had some of the best runs with friends who have or are experiencing the same symptoms as me. We share war stories and coping strategies. A run – and a problem – shared is a problem halved.

# Thermoregulation

Since hitting perimenopause, it feels like my body temperature runs a couple of degrees warmer, constantly, than it ever did before. The technical term for this is thermoregulation and, yes, it's mostly to do with fluctuations in hormones, namely the decline in oestrogen levels. Women talk about 'hot flashes' and I refer to myself as 'running hot'. Because that's what this feels like to me: as if I am a water boiler that is constantly on. For me and many others this increased body temperature impacts everything – sleep (leading to insomnia, which causes fatigue), the type of clothes we wear when running (they need to be not too tight and offer good air circulation) and the temperatures we feel comfortable running in (cold days are now my favourite).

> **HOW HORMONES AFFECT BODY TEMPERATURE**
>
> Here's the science bit – concentrate. Fluctuating hormone changes affect the hypothalamus, the part of the brain responsible for regulating body temperature. This leads to sensations of sudden warmth and sweating. When oestrogen levels fluctuate the hypothalamus becomes more sensitive to slight temperature changes, mistakenly perceiving the body as overheating.

But let's not put all the blame on oestrogen: some other hormones contribute, too, namely cortisol and adrenaline (stress hormones).

Thermoregulation triggers for female runners are:

- Warm weather
- Carbohydrate-heavy food
- Spicy food
- Caffeine (contained in a lot of sports products) and alcohol
- Tight running clothing
- High-effort running

Looking at all the causes and symptoms above it's no wonder that women in this phase of their lives find the act of running challenging. Here are some tips to help you manage your body temperature when learning to run:

**Wear loose, breathable clothing** – There is nothing worse than feeling constricted, as if your body cannot breathe. Wear loose-fitting T-shirts, jackets (if you even need one) and shorts. The only close-fitting things you really need to be wearing are your bra and trainers. Look for clothes that allow airflow, for your sweat to be able to be exposed to colder air, thus enabling your body to cool down. Remember to look for clothes that 'wick' sweat away (*see* p. 53).

**Layers** – Layering is your friend. Wear clothing layers that you can take off easily and either tie around your waist or store away in a small backpack or bum bag/fanny pack.

**Look out for triggers** – As you'll read in chapter 12, carbohydrates are a great source of quick-release energy but for many women – me in particular – overconsumption can exacerbate feelings of warmth. Be mindful of the effects that certain foods have on you and, if they increase symptoms, limit them. This is where your diary will come in useful. It has been found that foods that are rich in phytoestrogens (e.g. soy, flaxseeds, chickpeas, etc.) may help balance hormone levels. Caffeine – found in a lot of sports-marketed food and drinks – can cause sweats and overheating, so be mindful of how much you are ingesting.

**Keep running** – It *will not make your symptoms worse*. The type of running that I advocate in this book is about working mostly in your aerobic zone and running on 'feel' 80 per cent of the time. Running can reduce the frequency and intensity of hot flashes, running hot or even shivers (yes, some women experience shivers, too).

# Tendonitis issues

For the past few years, around the same month every year, my Achilles tendon starts to niggle. The first year I thought it was happening because of the trainers I was wearing, the undulating terrain I was running on, the fact I was carrying too much bodyweight and hadn't done enough strength training. So, I adjusted everything accordingly and, after a few months, it went away. But when the same thing happened around the same time the following year, and the year after, I became angry. 'What the hell is going on?' I thought and promptly booked an appointment with my physio. He said, 'Well of course, you're in perimenopause aren't you. That'll be contributing to it.'

What I didn't know then, and do now, is that women in perimenopause/menopause are more likely to experience tendon niggles. And guess what the number one issue is? Yep, you've guessed it: Achilles tendonitis.

Oestrogen plays an important role in maintaining the health and elasticity of tendons and ligaments, so its reduction during perimenopause can lead to structural and functional changes in these tissues. It also supports the production of collagen, a key protein in tendons that provides strength and flexibility. Falling levels = falling collagen, making tendons less elastic and more prone to micro-tears and overuse injuries. Oestrogen also helps to regulate our bodies' inflammatory response and supports tissue repair, so the fact that it's dropping in us means healing can be delayed and tendonitis can be increased.

But no one tells you that as a woman who runs or wants to run. Well, no one told me that until a man did. And now I am telling you.

Common tendonitis sites during perimenopause:

- Achilles tendon (ankles)
- Rotator cuff (shoulders)
- Tennis elbow (outer elbow)
- Golfer's elbow (inner elbow)
- Patellar tendon (knees)

So, what can we do to alleviate and manage tendonitis?

**Warm up and get mobile** – Always spend some time warming up and mobilising your body before the main session starts. This is so important. Please don't go into your session 'cold'. You need to ensure your body, and mind, is ready for exercise. I give much more direction on this in the Miles and Smiles chapter on page 212.

**Protein power** – Most of us do not know how much protein we should be consuming each day. Many of us don't get enough. Whether via real food or supplementation, there are a host of foods and products out there. Protein supports collagen synthesis and tissue repair, so however you choose to consume it, find a way that works for you. That might be through eggs, fish, meat or legumes, or it might be via a specially formulated protein shake or bar. The most important thing is that you get enough in. We will talk about nutrition more in chapter 12.

> #### HOW MUCH PROTEIN DO I NEED?
>
> Women in perimenopause should consider aiming to consume between 1.8–2.4 grams of protein per kilogram of bodyweight depending on activity levels.

**Hydration** – Are you drinking enough water? I know that, at times, I don't. But being hydrated helps to maintain elasticity. You are going to be increasing your exercise, so you need to stay hydrated. So, keep that water close by.

**Footwear** – We talked about trainers in chapter 4. Supportive, well-cushioned shoes help to reduce strain on tendons, especially during running.

And what if I feel a niggle?

**Manage it** – Use ice packs and over-the-counter anti-inflammatory medications if you feel any niggles.

**Rest it** – If you have a niggle and don't do anything about it, or continue to train thinking it'll go away, at some point you're probably going to have to stop running due to pain. Niggles are the body's way of telling you something isn't quite right – whether it's caused by a historical biological issue that has been exacerbated due to you starting to run or it is hormonal. Take the load off the affected area and rest. If the niggle doesn't calm down, or it comes back full throttle when you start running again, the next step is to seek some professional help.

**Get advice** – On the occasions I have experienced Achilles tendonitis I have had to follow a protocol, designed by my physiotherapist, of reduced load-bearing exercising (running) and increased non-load-bearing cross-training such as swimming and cycling. This has allowed me to maintain cardiovascular fitness while allowing the tendon a chance to settle down and/or repair. Alongside this cross-training I have also been prescribed strength and conditioning exercises focused on rehabilitation of the tendon. This protocol has meant a quick return to running and has given me the confidence to know I am not doing myself damage. It's at times like these that having a trusted expert to go to, for me a physiotherapist, is worth its weight in gold.

## Weight gain

'Thick thighs save lives!' That's what I used to say. I've always been an hourglass shape – DD boobs, small waist, decent childbearing hips and powerful thighs. I'll be honest with you and say – up until a few years ago – if I wanted to drop half a stone or a stone, I could do so easily. But a few years ago, something shifted. I was eating the same amount yet gaining a few pounds a month. I'd get angry with myself because I was still running the same average distances each week, still eating what I'd always eaten but the weight was piling on. Gradually, over a few months, I gained a stone. A bloody stone! I felt the weight mentally as well as physically when

I was running and blamed myself for a lack of willpower and all those other negative things we like to tell ourselves.

But it wasn't due to my lack of self-discipline or my greediness for wanting to lick my plate clean. That extra stone was the gift perimenopause gave me that I didn't ask for. The hormonal rollercoaster ride that we are on – and the symptoms associated with it – leads to weight gain. And we often see that around our midriff. There are multiple reasons for this. If you are fatigued or aren't sleeping well, you're more likely to reach for high-calorie foods. Low oestrogen reduces your sensitivity to insulin, leading to increased fat storage. A slower metabolism, which comes with ageing, means that we might eat the same amount of calories but gain weight.

It's not your fault. It's part of the process. But what can we do?

In short, an amalgamation of all the things above and doing them consistently. Eating well, running on feel, doing strength and conditioning work, running with other women going through the same thing. All of it.

But the one thing I want to remind you is this – and it's SO important: no matter what your size or how many extra pounds you believe you are carrying, you can run. Lighter does not mean better or faster and it *certainly* doesn't mean stronger. Running is for every one of you. No matter your shape or size.

## Get some R&R

There's no getting around it, as we age, recovery from any form of exercise – running included – can take longer. In perimenopause all the hormone changes and symptoms we experience contribute to the time it takes for us to feel ready to go again. I know it takes me so much longer to recover from a particularly challenging run than it ever used to. That's why rest and recovery is super important because it's in this phase that we get stronger. We rest to build.

When it comes to the running plan that I have designed in the Miles and Smiles chapter on page 212, it is aimed at ensuring good recovery.

**Rest days** – I encourage you to take rest days in between your run sessions to allow for recovery, with a caveat that if you need more time, take it. You know your body. You know how it feels and that it is responding to the stimulus that you are placing on it. Recover well.

**Quality, not quantity** – You do not need to do five sessions a week, or four, or even three if you don't want to. On my C25K plan, the minimum amount of run sessions I ask you to do, per week, is two – because I focus on quality, not quantity. During the sessions I prescribe, we will focus on different 'quality' elements (and they're a surprise for now) so you will get all you need from each session without running metaphorically into a wall.

**Listen to your body** – What Shirley the runner down the road does is none of your business. She's not you. In chapter 5 I talked about the importance of running on feel, of listening to your body and all of the cues that it gives you in terms of its energy and recovery needs. If you ignore how you feel when you run, you will not enjoy this process. If you do not take time to recover, or compare the time it takes you to recover against the woman down the road/online, you will not enjoy this process and, in addition to that, you might get injured.

## Supplemental support during the perimenopause

### Iron
In my conversations with both Cath and Renee – who you will hear from more in chapter 12 – both experts discussed with me the importance of iron supplementation for female runners who are in perimenopause

and menopause. Low iron levels can cause you to experience a range of symptoms such as persistent fatigue even after rest, muscle weakness, breathlessness and injury.

> **DEALING WITH ANAEMIA**
>
> 'I've been anaemic for most of my adult life and have suffered with heavy and painful periods. I started taking contraception 17 years ago, which means they did become less painful, but I still sometimes had heavy and prolonged bleeding. I take prescription-strength iron as a prophylaxis and, if I need to, I take hormonal medication to stop the bleeding completely for a few months. When I become anaemic, I suffer badly with low energy and can almost fall asleep when I sit down at any time of day. Low iron also affects my anxiety. The panic attack-like symptoms always completely disappear once I take my iron again.'

For female runners, some of the ways that iron is lost in the body is through heavy or irregular periods, sweating, inadequate diet (focusing on carbohydrates to the detriment of iron-rich foods), and the body's inability to absorb iron due to hormone changes that reduce stomach acid, thus impairing iron absorption.

Symptoms associated with low iron, such as fatigue, shortness of breath and dizziness, are something to be mindful of and, personally, I have been caught out a few times in my running life. I've requested a blood test to confirm my iron levels were low, and I have been prescribed a course of iron tablets, which has put me right and made me feel like a new woman.

Other things that might help lessen symptoms of low iron include:

**Eating iron-rich foods** – Include easy-to-absorb iron-rich foods in your diet, such as lean red meat, liver, poultry, fish and eggs as well as dark leafy greens, kale, chickpeas and quinoa. You can also enhance the absorption of iron by pairing food with vitamin C sources, such as citrus fruits, bell peppers and tomatoes.

**Taking iron supplements** – I took a course of ferrous sulphate as advised by my doctor. But if you have a sensitive stomach, you might need a slower-release iron supplement. Talk to your GP.

**Manage heavy or irregular periods** – To manage my flooding I was advised to have a Mirena coil inserted. This helped lessen flooding and also, as a bonus, it provides progestin – a synthetic form of progesterone – which helps balance my fluctuating hormones too. Again, consult your doctor.

Keep track of symptoms that could indicate iron deficiency (see above) and – if you are concerned – go and get checked out.

## Supplements for menopause

Research shows that many women have had success in using supplements and herbal remedies to manage specific symptoms, and potential deficiencies, caused by menopause such as insomnia, mood regulation, anxiety, bone strength, etc. These supplements and remedies include but are not limited to:

**Vitamin D** – Most of us need to take vitamin D for at least some of the year. There are of course some countries in the world that get far more sunlight than we do here in the UK but, even so, vitamin D supplementation is a must in the autumn and winter months.

**Calcium** – Beneficial during menopause primarily to maintain bone health and reduce the risk of osteoporosis. It helps to reduce the loss of bone mineral, making bones stronger and less prone to fracture.

**Magnesium** – This supports bone density, muscle relaxation, sleep and mood. It can also help reduce cramps, headaches and anxiety and improve muscle recovery.

**Collagen** – This helps maintain skin elasticity, joint health and bone strength. But remember, the type and dose are really important. Bovine collagen is the most supported, with scientific studies stating doses of 10–15mg are necessary to make any difference. So, ensure that you are looking at the labels closely.

**Evening primrose oil and starflower oil** – Studies show that perimenopausal women who have used these herbal remedies have reported a reduction in breast tenderness.

**Black cohosh** – This can help reduce hot flashes, night sweats and mood swings.

**Red clover** – This contains phytoestrogens that may mimic oestrogen and alleviate menopausal symptoms.

**Sage** – Aids sleep.

When it comes to over-the-counter and herbal remedies that you can take to alleviate your symptoms, the list is endless. And, as we are all individual, some will work for us and some won't. I am not a doctor and the decisions that you make must be yours based on your lifestyle and what works for you. Speak to a pharmacist, doctor, or holistic practitioner for advice on specific doses to support your menopause journey.

As a female who runs, all I can do is share with you what has worked for me. I use magnesium. I have a scoop of collagen in my coffee every morning. I ingest iron in food when I can and, when I need more, I take a supplement. And I also use hormone replacement therapy (HRT). This might not be a good combination for Shirley, the runner down the road, but it works for me.

## Hormone replacement therapy

There are so many books, podcasts, videos and experts much more experienced than I who can tell you the positives and negatives of HRT. I feel it would be remiss of me to even try to go into the ins and outs of why you should or shouldn't take it. All I can do is tell you that I started using HRT a few years ago and my symptoms have been reduced. They have not gone completely but they are manageable and do not seriously impact my busy life, or my running. I am OK, for now. Every morning, I rub my HRT gel into a part of my body, I sip my collagen-boosted coffee, pop my iron tablet and antidepressant and I live on to run another day. Maybe that works for you, too? Maybe it doesn't. But, please, find what does and know that running will be a key ally in your toolbox of 'stuff that does work' during this phase.

## And what about after?! (Menopause)

Is it wrong for me to say that I long for a specific day? That day when it has been a year since the date of my last period and I can finally say I am in menopause. I am not scared of it. I am ready for it. Are you there? If so, and you are thinking about taking up running, then I want to help you know what to do. I therefore asked Dr Cath about what women who start running in menopause need to be mindful of.

She said: 'As the roller coaster of oestrogen levels start to settle, many symptoms will ease as well. Most women find that they settle into a more predictable state. That state might include higher levels of anxiety than in the past, continued aches and pains and feeling hotter (or colder!), for example. But the roller coaster tends to go away.

'If women are still on HRT, then they can rest assured that their bones are still being protected. Women aged 60 and over tend to find that they'll need less oestrogen but, if you don't want to come off it completely, you don't have to. There's no maximum length of time to be on HRT.'

When it comes to running in menopause you may well still experience aches and pains, hot flashes or feeling as if you are running hot but, for most, these will be lessened. However, as I have said before, we are all unique. Cath confirms this: 'I see women in their 70s and 80s who are still getting hot.'

If you are in menopause then all the tips associated with management of perimenopause symptoms above will help you, no matter how old you are.

However, there are some additional things that women who are starting to run in menopause need to be aware of.

## Vulval and vaginal health

If you are menopausal and have been for some time then you might be more prone to experiencing some leaking. Pelvic floor exercises (*see* p. 192) are so important, so please don't forget to do them. You do not have to put up with leaking. You can still work to keep things in check.

## Treat your vagina like you treat your face

If you do not moisturise your vagina then it can be prone to irritation and tearing. Vaginal oestrogen is a number one recommendation from Dr Cath and there are ranges of preparations for internal use that come with applicators (pessaries such as Vagirux and creams that contain estriol). There are also ranges of branded vaginal moisturisers that are for internal use.

For external use, normal moisturisers such as Aveeno or other non-perfumed products are OK. Cath recommends oatmeal-based ones. Estriol creams and Vagirux, mentioned above, can also be used externally.

Think about it. You moisturise your face to keep it soft, elastic, radiant and – for some of us – youthful! Why not your vagina? Treat it well.

## Urinary/bowel urgency

I know that I am not the only one to experience the sudden urgent need to pee or poo while out on a run. And I know that it is one of the key things that women worry about. 'What if I need to go to the toilet and there is nowhere to go nearby?' It's part of the reason that I love trail running, as there are lots of bushes! It's also why we discuss the importance of giving your body some time to let food settle before you go on a run and finding foods that don't irritate your bowel. Also make sure you use the toilet – even if you don't feel you need it – before you run.

## Bone health

Thinking about your bone health is important. There are websites that allow you to do your own simple bone assessment. By answering a few questions, you will be advised whether you might need a bone (DEXA) scan or not. For women, using a resource such as this gives us a sense of control without having to take a trip to the doctor. Running and strength and conditioning helps to improve bone health. But if your starting point is that you have some osteoporosis (weak and brittle bones), or osteopenia (low bone mass), it's important to know about the risks associated with that and whether you will be more prone to injury.

> **WHAT IS A DEXA SCAN?**
>
> A DEXA scan measures your bone mineral density – which indicates how strong and dense your bones are – using low-dose X-rays. It helps to diagnose or assess the risk of osteoporosis and other bone-related conditions. The scan is normally performed in a hospital or radiology clinic.

## Riding the roller coaster

This phase of life is like riding a roller coaster. One day you're up and the next you're down with heightened anxiety around 'What the hell's next?' But just like we are asked to do at a theme park, we've got to strap in and trust that we will get through the ride. When it comes to managing symptoms associated with perimenopause and menopause, I urge you to really take time to listen to your body. Ensure that, if symptoms are stopping you living the life you want to, you get the tests you need (such as measuring your iron levels; there is no point getting a blood test to measure your hormone levels since these fluctuate so much). Do your research, speak to other women going through it, and seek expert advice on HRT and other resources that can support you. And please know that learning to run is a positive thing that you can do that will support your journey and alleviate, rather than negatively affect, symptoms.

CHAPTER 11

# Stronger than yesterday

If there is one thing that I would gently urge – or annoyingly poke – you to do alongside your run practice, it's some strength and conditioning (S&C). The benefits for you as a new runner far outweigh any perceived negatives. And I promise you, I am not asking you to go and 'lift heavy' at the local gym. Everything that I and my own physiotherapist, Ed, prescribe in this chapter can be done in 20 minutes at home, with – if you want to – items that you have in the cupboard.

So, what is S&C and why should you do it?

> **FEEL THE POWER!**
>
> 'Strength training has had a huge impact on my running. It has helped me to improve how long I can run for, my posture and how stable I feel. I also think it's actually made me much more powerful when I am trying to run fast and when climbing hills, too!'

## What is strength and conditioning?

Strength and conditioning is a form of training that involves the repetition of a variety of exercises that focuses on developing your body's strength, power and mobility and enhances its recovery.

When it comes to running, the impact force that our bodies absorb when our foot hits the ground is two to three times our bodyweight, so, to really enjoy the journey of running, S&C is a key cross-training component to developing your running resilience.

The benefits of S&C training include:

- **Injury prevention** – As a runner, having strong muscles will help your body absorb force (how much force comes back up through the body) that can damage your joints. Having strong muscles can also prevent you experiencing overuse injuries in the lower back and legs. Strength training can also help to improve posture and includes techniques that reduce the risk of injury when you get tired.
- **Improved performance** – Strength training will help to improve your power, your speed, your endurance and your agility. It will also help you to use the oxygen you inhale more efficiently due to an increase of 'powerhouse' cells that enable your muscles to use oxygen more efficiently. It'll also stimulate the growth of capillaries around your muscle fibres, which will help to improve oxygen delivery to your working muscles and get rid of lactic acid.
- **Greater bone density** – This is an important one for you to remember if you are perimenopausal or menopausal: strength training helps increase bone density, which can prevent osteoporosis later in life. Pair it with running and you could become bulletproof!
- **Increased endurance** – Strength training can help improve your cardiovascular fitness and muscular endurance, which in turn helps to increase your running endurance (being able to run for a longer period of time).
- **More muscle mass** – Strength and conditioning programmes can help build muscle mass, which can improve performance and reduce the risk of injury. It also improves insulin sensitivity, resulting in fewer glucose spikes and a reduced chance of getting type 2 diabetes.
- **Better co-ordination** – It will improve the connection between your brain and your muscles, which will make your running a lot easier and reduce your chances of injury.

- **Improved mental health** – It increases serotonin release, which can improve mood and reduce stress.
- **Greater flexibility** – It improves flexibility and mobility.
- **More positive body image** – Being strong really does make you feel and look great!

I know that there are some common reasons why lots of women do not engage in strength and conditioning. Do any of these sound like you?

'I don't know what exercises to do.'

'I don't have time to fit it in.'

'I don't want to join a gym.'

'I don't know how to use the machines at the gym and the weights room looks really intimidating.'

'I don't want to get bigger.'

Let's address these concerns head-on.

## I don't know what exercises to do

Of course, right now, you don't know what to do. There are hundreds of different exercises out there, thousands in fact, and it's overwhelming. I get it. I understand. There are different exercises that focus on different connective tissues, muscles and joints and – unless you are a qualified professional – how are you to know which ones to pick? That's not your job.

Let me guide you through some tried-and-tested exercises that have been proven to help female runners just like you.

## I don't have time to fit it in

You've got a busy life. You're juggling family, friends, a job, the dog, the cat, the house. You've bought this book because you want to try running and now I am asking, gently advising, that you incorporate strength and conditioning training, too?!

'Give me a break!' I hear you say.

My response: 'I'm giving you this advice so you *don't* break.'

I would never advocate anything that didn't work. This will work. This will help you. Trust me. All I ask is for 20 minutes a week (minimum) of your time. Yes, 20 minutes. I'll say it again. I am not asking you to spend any more than 20 minutes one or two times per week on your strength and conditioning.

## I don't want to join a gym

You don't have to. Not until you want to. If ever. I know from talking to women that gym spaces – especially for those who have not used them before – can be intimidating. The people, the equipment, the music, the cost. All of these things combined can create a culture of fear, of imposter syndrome and increased barriers to you accessing them. Gyms profit off a massive influx of new members each January and bank on almost 50 per cent of these people never coming back (but forgetting to cancel their direct debit).

The exercises below are designed to be done in whatever space you currently have access to. If that's the kitchen, so be it. If that's floor space at the gym you are a member of, so be it. All you need is you (and me to guide you).

## I don't know how to use the machines at the gym and the weights room is intimidating

The reason that there are fitness instructors in charge of gym spaces is to assist you. Not to stand around looking pretty or spotting (holding weights) for their friends or favourite clients who are there.

As part of any gym induction, you should be shown how to use the gym equipment and, more often than not, be prescribed a programme tailored to your needs. If this has not happened then I would question the safety procedures of the gym you are a member of. If there is specific equipment that you feel you do not understand, speak to a member of staff and – if you need to – book an appointment. You are paying for a service.

In many gyms there are often 'free weights' rooms or dedicated spaces. This is where you will often see people who look 'stacked' (a common term for very muscular people) and who can often be heard making funny noises when they are lifting heavy weights. Unfortunately, in this age of social media one-upmanship, these are also the spaces where you will see people posing in front of full-length mirrors to get the best lighting angles to define their bulging muscles or six-pack stomach for social media 'likes'.

I am a confident woman and even I can be intimidated, and annoyed, trying to work out in gym spaces but, again, if you are paying for a gym membership then this space is as much yours as it is theirs and a polite 'Are you using this piece of equipment?' is a gentle signal for them to move on. No one, no matter how they look, has a monopoly on this public space.

## I don't want to get bigger

There is a long-standing myth that strength and conditioning training – and lifting weights in particular – will make you become bulky. This untruth has led to many women never trying to pick up a weight, which has had a detrimental effect on their fitness, muscle mass and confidence and has further reinforced harmful stereotypes and outdated beauty standards about who should and who should not participate in strength and conditioning.

Please know that how your muscles grow is highly individual to you and is influenced by genetics, diet, training intensity and hormones. Also know that testosterone plays a significant role in muscle growth and, since we have lower levels of this hormone than men, and it decreases as we age, our capacity for developing larger, bulky muscles is limited.

The strength – training exercises below are all about making you a more resilient runner, not becoming a bodybuilder. This will result, over time, in a toned and strong, not oversized, build – making you a more resilient runner.

### I WISH I HAD STARTED 10 YEARS AGO!

'I am 54 this year and am currently in perimenopause. I have to admit, I have been having a real time of it. Last year I took up strength training and it has been so invaluable. I enlisted the help of a personal trainer to make sure I was doing it right. It just makes my running feel so much easier. I feel so much stronger! I just wish I'd started doing it 10 years ago!'

# Running resilience in 20 minutes

What if I told you that, if you committed just 20 minutes a week, it would make you a more resilient runner? A stronger runner. A more mobile and flexible runner. Would you believe me? And, more important than that, would you be willing to try it?

I've been working with the most amazing physiotherapist for the last few years. I found him through a friend, and he has helped me to navigate countless injuries and niggles effectively and safely, which has meant I have been able to continue running. His name is Ed and I brought him on board for this chapter, to offer his professional insight.

Ed believes, as I do, that runners' strength and conditioning is about 'quality not quantity'. And, when it comes to integrating strength and conditioning training into your weekly schedule, that's what we want you to focus on.

We believe that to make the best use of your time there are three key exercises that focus on lower body, upper body, core and plyometrics (bouncing and jumping) that you can start to incorporate that will make you a more resilient runner.

Ed's experience in prescribing exercises to his clients as a physio mimic mine as a personal trainer in that 'too much too soon leads to overwhelm' and 'overwhelm leads to inactivity'. So, in this chapter, we're all about the KISS (keep it simple, stupid) method.

Below, we have stipulated three exercises for each category. Each category should take you no longer than 20 minutes to complete. We want you to focus on *form* and *feel*.

## How should it feel?

When it comes to strength and conditioning training, the key word is 'challenge'. If you want to build strength and, ultimately, the capacity of a muscle(s) then you have to challenge it.

What should it feel like to challenge your muscles during a strength and conditioning session? Well, in the words of Ed: 'It should be tiring, not painful. It should not be completely exhausting to the point of failure ('point of failure' is when you can't actually perform the action/exercise).

You should be able to complete the required repetitions of the exercise in a set and think, "Yes, I am glad that is done. It was hard and I am feeling tired."'

> **JARGON BUSTER: REPETITIONS AND SETS**
>
> A repetition (rep) is the number of times you do an exercise in unbroken sequence (e.g. 10 squats one after the other).
>
> A set is a required number of reps being done in unbroken sequence. For example, 1 x 10 reps (squats). That means 1 unbroken set of 10 squats.

## Delayed onset muscle soreness (DOMS)

DOMS is something that you will likely experience as part of your running journey – more so as a new or returning runner. You'll experience it as muscle pain and stiffness that you can start to feel 24–72 hours after you run or strength train. DOMS will have you moving slower than you normally do and those activities that might have seemed easy yesterday will feel much harder when you add DOMS to the mix. DOMS happen because, each time you exercise, tiny muscle fibres get damaged. But please don't worry, that is part of the process! Your body works to repair these muscle fibres, and, in the process, gets stronger. The soreness that you experience should go away on its own, but you can help by continuing to gently move, stretch, eat (protein-rich foods – see chapter 12), hydrate and – my favourite – soak those muscles in a warm Epsom salt bath.

If you are still experiencing pain and soreness five to seven days after exercising, you may want to seek expert support, such as a physiotherapist, as it could be a sign of injury.

## You can do anything for 20 minutes!

For strength and conditioning training to be successful, it's about creating time for it. Look at your life currently. Where in your day would be the easiest place for you to carve out 20 minutes? In the morning?

Later in the evening? After the school run? I know it's not possible for everyone but, if you can create regular space for your 20-minute session then it will be easier to convert it into a habit – remember chapter 2?! And we're all about creating habits.

## Be patient

Truth bomb time: you are not going to see, visually, immediate physical changes when you start strength and conditioning training. It may take six weeks or longer for you to feel *any* physical benefits of the 20-minute routine(s) you will be practising but, trust me, those feelings of strength, of power, of endurance *will* come.

My experience in coaching women, and doing my own strength and conditioning, has shown me that *consistency breeds habit and habit breeds results*. And, for female runners, I have had much joy in witnessing that light-bulb moment when they suddenly 'feel' stronger when running.

Gentle progression and adaptation – taking it slowly, focusing on quality and allowing the body adequate recovery time to adapt – is crucial to remember when seeking to get stronger as a runner.

Going 'beast mode' for seven days a week is not a discipline of coaching I teach. It is in allowing our bodies the time to adapt to the training stresses that we place on it that we get stronger. That we become more resilient female runners.

Ed backs this up: 'The work that you do in those early stages lays such great foundations that, when a woman has that "aha" moment, it really gives an injection of motivation to stick with the strength and conditioning training as a component to their running. Patience is key.'

## Bodyweight is brilliant

To start to integrate strength training into your life all you need is *you*. Believe me, you don't need to spend hundreds of pounds on expensive kit to get started. Your wonderful body will provide all of the resistance you need. I don't want you to worry about 'how to hold this' and 'where to place that'. By keeping things simple, you will think more about how your body is moving in accordance with the exercise cues I give you. Let's not overcomplicate this. As you will see, I have picked a selection of exercises that rely solely on you.

Let's get started!

> ### A NOTE ON SHOES FOR STRENGTH TRAINING
>
> Ideally, you should wear trainers that have a flat sole and not too much cushioning when doing strength and conditioning. Or, even better, go barefoot or train in your socks! This is so that you can feel the floor more, which will help you balance, and they will also help you transfer force from your muscles. Squishy, shock-absorbing running trainers can be unstable, and they are designed to absorb force, which will negatively affect your strength training.

## The exercises

In the table on p. 187 are names, reps, sets and suggested rest periods for four groups of my favourite simple but effective strength and conditioning exercises. But first you need to learn how to do them.

# Lower body

## SQUAT

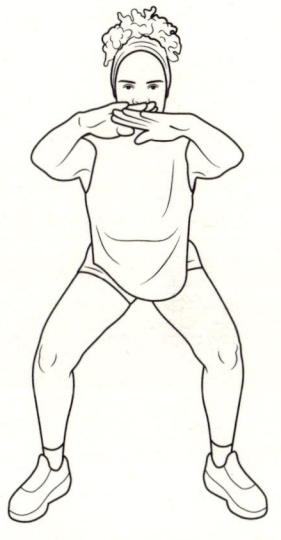

Think about technique. Start with your feet relatively wide, at least shoulder-width apart and maybe even a little bit wider. Your toes should be pointing out to (if you were looking at a clock) the 11 and 1 o'clock positions. Drop down so that your hips come below your knees to get your glutes (bum muscles) involved in the action, otherwise this can become a very quad-dominant exercise. And don't get me wrong, that's OK, but – for this exercise – we want to target the bum.

As you lower down into the squat position keep an eye on your knees; the aim is not to let them collapse inwards. And when lowering, think about the action of you sitting back into a chair, rather than going into a crouch. You can even place a chair behind you and gently lower onto it if that feels good to start off with. Your arms should be held out in front of you, straight and parallel with your shoulders.

A key point to note is that if you cannot achieve this squat position without your heels rising then please put something under your heels. A couple of books about an inch thick would do the trick. By adding this small support for your heels most people will find that they are able to achieve the desired position by being able to drop down deep enough to make the exercise more effective.

Squats are amazing. They are such a versatile exercise and can be progressed easily by holding something in front of your body as you drop down. Items at home such as a bag for life filled with bottles of milk, bags of sugar or a small child(!) will suffice! Or choose an easier route and order a set of dumbbells or a kettlebell on the internet. I bought my mum a set of dumbbells for Christmas once as a replacement for the traditional Ferrero Rocher. She told me she loves them!

## SPLIT SQUAT

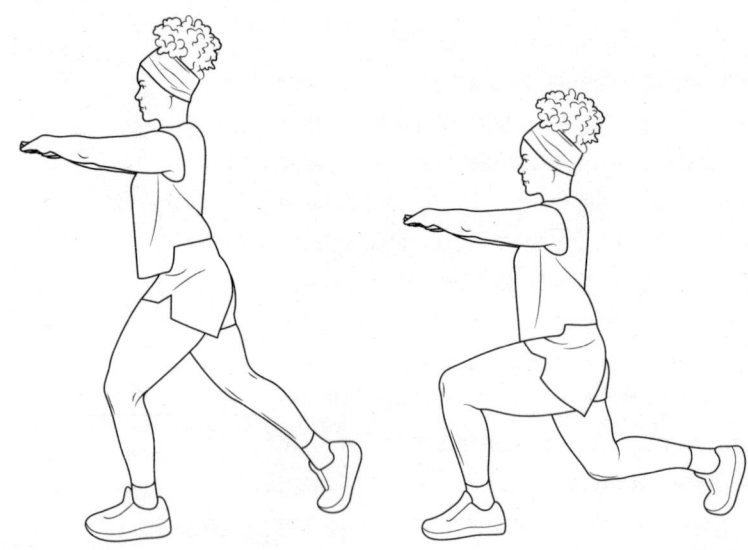

You will be working similar muscles to those that you are using in the regular squat, but by being in a split stance position you will be mimicking the way that you run (your running mechanics) a little bit more. Again, technique is super important.

   To perform the exercise, stand upright with your feet hip-distance apart. Take a step back with your right foot, keeping your left foot forwards. Your right foot should be positioned a few feet behind you with your toes pointing slightly forwards, but make sure your left foot is flat on the ground. When you are ready to lower, keep your chest up and slowly lower your body, bending at your left knee and allowing your right knee to come down towards the floor. Ensure that your left knee stays aligned over your left ankle and doesn't extend past your toes. Lower your body until your left thigh is parallel to the ground or slightly lower and your right knee is hovering just above the floor. To rise, press through your left heel to return to your starting position. Keep the movement slow and controlled. Repeat the sequence on the other side.

## SLOUCH

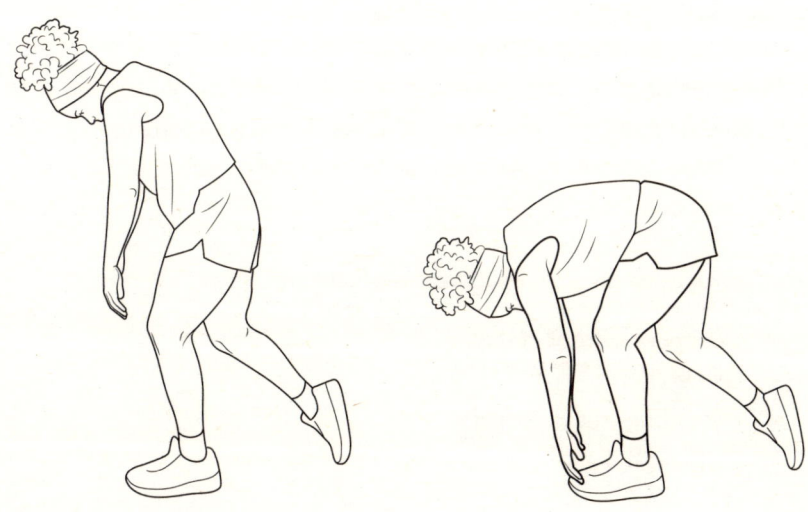

This exercise is designed to help what we call the 'posterior chain' – that is the calf, hamstrings and the glutes. The aim here is to get all these muscles working well together as a unit to help improve the mechanics of the legs while we run.

If you are working on the left leg, start by standing on just the left foot, so all of your weight is going through the left side, then put the right foot down just behind the left. The back leg is simply there to act as a balancing post – 99 per cent of your weight should stay on the front foot throughout. Bend the left knee to a maximum of 20 degrees – you are aiming to keep the knee at this angle throughout the entire exercise. Next, relax your back and shoulders as much as you can, aiming to keep the upper body relaxed throughout the entire exercise. The reason for this is to force the muscles in the leg to do the work without any help from the back leg. Keeping your weight towards the front half of the right foot, slowly reach your fingertips down towards the floor without letting the knee bend any further and keeping the back relaxed throughout. Once you are down as far as you feel you can go, press down into the ground through the front of the left foot and then slowly bring yourself back up, again keeping the back as relaxed as you possibly can. Once you get to a point where your hands are level with that left knee, go straight back down again and repeat on the other side.

You should feel this working predominantly in your calf muscle but also in the hamstrings and the glutes. It shouldn't take many repetitions to feel some fatigue in the muscles of the leg. Try to go slowly to maintain control of the position of the knee and to keep the muscles under duress as much as possible.

What lower body muscle groups are we focusing on?

- Quadriceps (front of thigh)
- Glutes (bum)
- Hamstrings (back of thigh)
- Calf (lower leg)

## Upper body

To run well, we need our arms, chest, upper back and shoulders to be strong and involved. Pay them some attention and they will improve your running!

Let's talk about push-ups, which for me, and many women, can be a bugbear. Why? Because sometimes doing just a few, and maintaining the correct form while doing so, can seem like such an effort. This is where it is important to give yourself some grace and start small. The good news is that to start to practise push-ups, you don't even need to get on the floor!

### UPPING THE ANTE

'I used to neglect my upper body but now, after incorporating exercises into my strength training, I feel a lot stronger when running. It feels like my arms are now helping to move me forwards faster.'

## WALL PUSH-UP

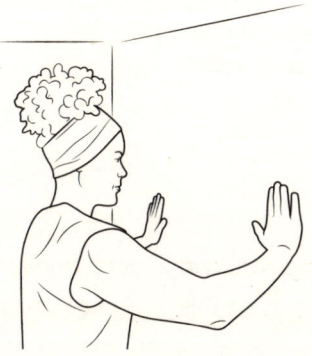

You can start off by performing a push-up while standing and pushing against a wall. This will help to reduce the intensity of the exercise and enable you to feel the muscles that you are looking to engage. To do it, stand facing a wall, about an arm's length away. Place your hands on the wall at shoulder height and slightly wider than shoulder-width apart. Point your fingers up with your palms flat against the wall. Step your feet back slightly so your body is at a slight incline and keep them hip-width apart for balance. Engage your core and keep your body in a straight line from head to heels. Inhale and bend your elbows while you slowly lean your chest against the wall. Keep your elbows at a 45-degree angle from your body and stop when your chest is close to the wall. Now exhale as you push yourself back to the starting position, straightening your arms. Repeat the movement.

## MODIFIED PUSH-UP

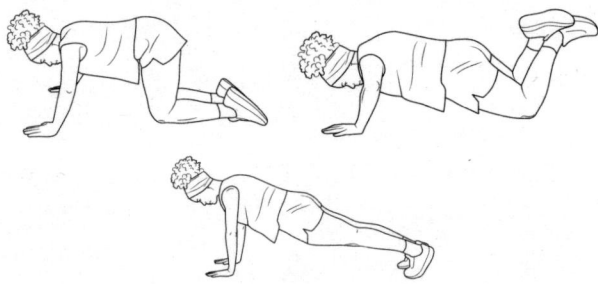

This modified push-up will work your chest, shoulders, back and triceps. To do it, get into a table-top position with your knees on the ground and your hands placed slightly wider than shoulder-width apart. Ensure that your wrists are directly under your shoulders. Engage your core to maintain your body's stability. Spread your fingers wide and press your palms firmly into the ground to push yourself up into the starting position. Your elbows can be slightly out to the sides, or you can tuck them closer to your body. Then inhale as you bend your elbows to lower your chest towards the ground, keeping your elbows at about a 45-degree angle relative to your body. Exhale as you push up through your palms and raise your body back to the starting position. Really focus on engaging your chest, shoulders and triceps. Keep your body in a straight line from your knees to your shoulders; don't let that bum rise up! Repeat for the required number of reps.

**To progress to a half plank press-up** – Move your knees further back and drop your hips so that there is a straight line from your knees to your shoulders. Engage your core to maintain stability and perform the push-up. Once you feel stronger repeating the repetitions in this position, progress to a full push-up.

**To progress to a full push-up** – Start in a full plank position (see p. 178) with your knees off the floor. Now, place your palms on the floor to the side of you and push your body up until your arms are almost straight. Lower your chest as far to the floor as you are able without losing position, then exhale and push back up, keeping your core engaged and your body straight.

## STANDING DUMBBELL ARM SWING

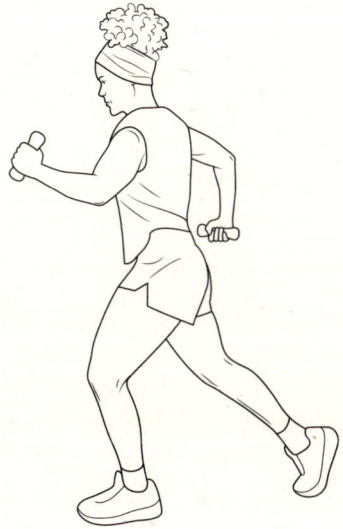

This one works your triceps and biceps and improves your running arm action. Hold a can of beans (or a similar home product) or weights, if you have them, in each hand and stand with one foot in front of the other in a split stance (one leg behind the other) to help you balance. Swing your arms back and forth, alternately, and mimic the action of your running, keeping your elbows bent at around 90 degrees. Make sure that you have brought your elbow all the way back before moving your arm forwards again. Your arms should be parallel to each other as they swing back and forth; don't allow them to cross over your body. Doing this exercise in front of a mirror can sometimes help you understand the technique and minimise core rotation. Engage your core to keep you stable. Repeat for the desired number of repetitions.

## SINGLE-ARM DUMBBELL ROW

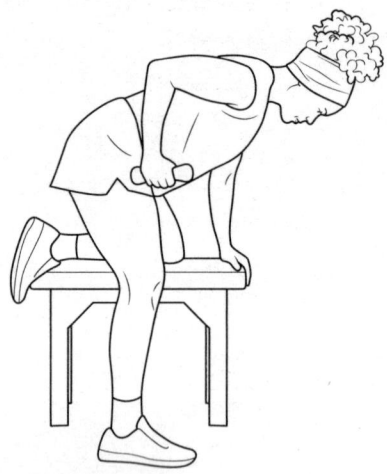

This is a great one for your back muscles as well as your biceps. You'll need some form of bench, firm sofa or even a coffee table to kneel on. If you have a light dumbbell – or something around the house that weighs 1kg (2 or 3lb), such as a 1-litre bottle of water – grab that, too. To do it, place your right knee on top of the bench and bend forwards from your waist until your back is flat and parallel to the floor. Place your right hand on the bench for support. Use your left hand to pick up the weight and keep your palm facing towards your torso and your elbows in. Now gently pull the weight up to the side of your chest, keeping your elbow in and close to your side. Lower it back down to the start position and repeat for the desired number of repetitions. Once done, repeat on the other side, changing legs so that your left leg and left hand are on top of the bench and your right arm does the work. Remember to keep your elbows close to your body and your back flat. Try not to twist your upper body during the exercise.

**To progress** – As you get stronger, increase the weight (you may need to buy some dumbbells at this point, but they're well worth the investment!).

## Core

If you want to remind yourself of the importance of your core in terms of running technique, what muscles make it up and how to activate it then – rather than me explaining it again to you here – I advise you to turn to p. 34.

Here are some exercises that will help you to strengthen this important group of muscles.

# HALF PLANK

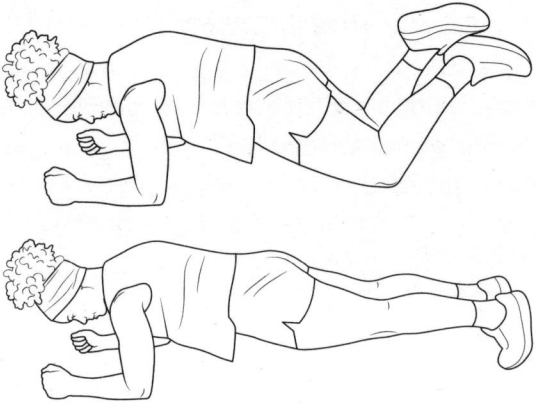

Planks are great core exercises. They are static (in that they don't involve any movement within the exercise itself) but, due to the way they can be varied, they are simple to learn and, once you feel stronger, easy to progress (make a bit more challenging). A half plank is a great option for beginners.

Here's how to do it. Get on the ground and start on all fours, placing your hands directly under your shoulders and your knees under your hips. Now lower to your forearms, keeping your elbows directly under your shoulders. Extend your body by stepping your feet back slightly so that your body forms a straight line from your head to your knees (which are touching the ground). Now engage your core, keeping your abdominal muscles tight and intentionally avoiding arching or sagging your lower back. Aim to hold for 20 seconds to start and remember to breathe steadily. To come out of the plank, bring your knees back to table-top position and rest.

**To progress to a forearm plank** – Once you feel stronger, to progress from a half plank to a forearm plank you need to repeat the movement above but, as an extra step, walk your feet back further and then bring your knees off the ground. You are aiming for your body to be in a straight line from your heels to your head. Again, keep that core engaged with no arching or sagging of the lower back. Once in position, hold for as long as you are able to without losing form.

## WHAT IS FORM?

'Form' refers to the proper technique and body positions that we use when performing an exercise. Making sure to keep good form will minimise injury and maximise the benefits the exercise gives you. Ensuring good form is almost as important as getting through each exercise. It's about quality, not quantity.

## DEAD BUG

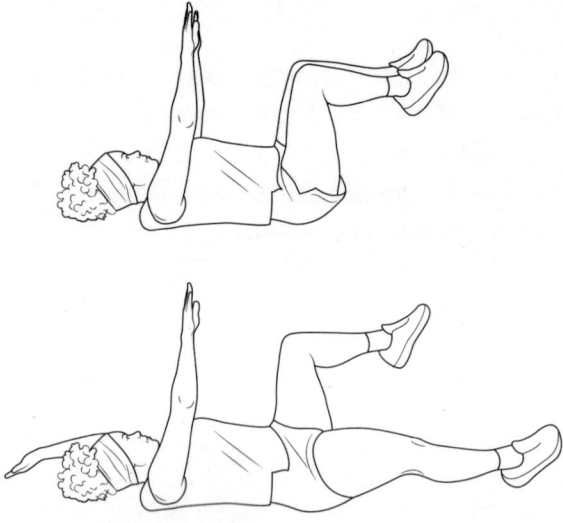

A dead bug is a great core exercise for runners. It is a dynamic core strength movement that, at the same time as working your core, also improves co-ordination and mimics the running movement (due to you working one shoulder at the same time as the opposite hip). To do it, lie on your back with your arms extended straight up towards the ceiling and then raise your legs so that your knees are bent at a 90-degree angle with your shins parallel to the floor. Gently press your lower back into the floor by tilting your pelvis. To help you understand what this feels like, place your hands under your lower back – palms down on the floor – and tilt your pelvis up until you feel your back making contact with the top of your hands. Remove your hands and continue to fill the gap. Ensuring this contact will help maintain your neutral spine – a position where your spine is neither excessively arched nor overly rounded, which allows optimal posture, stability and movement efficiency – and engage your core. Slowly lower your right arm overhead to the floor behind you and your left leg towards the floor while keeping your lower back pressed into the ground. Go as low as you can *without* arching your back, then return to the starting position by bringing them back up. Now switch sides by lowering your left arm and right leg. Continue for the required number of repetitions.

## OBLIQUE TWIST

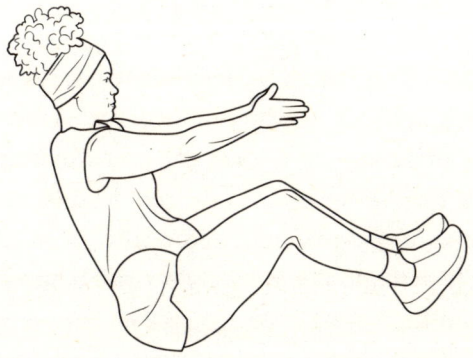

This is a great exercise for targeting your oblique muscles and improving core stability. Your oblique muscles are at the side of your abdomen and run between your lower ribs and pelvis. To do it, sit on the floor with your knees bent and your feet flat on the ground. Lean back slightly, keeping your back straight and your core engaged. Place your hands together in an outstretched prayer position in front of your chest. Rotate your upper body to the right, keeping your hips facing forwards. You should feel the side of your body tightening (this means your obliques are contracting). To keep your legs stable, focus on using your core to control your twist. Rotate your upper body back to the centre, then twist to the left, following the same movement pattern. Continue alternating the twist for the required number of repetitions.

## Plyometrics

I am keen for you to try some jumping. I should warn you – if you have dogs or kids around, they might want to get involved. I tell you this from experience!

Jumping is one of the most underutilised exercises for improving your running technique. Think about it: every time we are out running, we are basically pushing our bodies forwards by jumping from one foot to the other. The better your body gets at this, and you can start by practising some of the exercises below, the more your muscles will respond positively to it and the more power you'll have in each step you take when out running.

## JUMP SQUAT

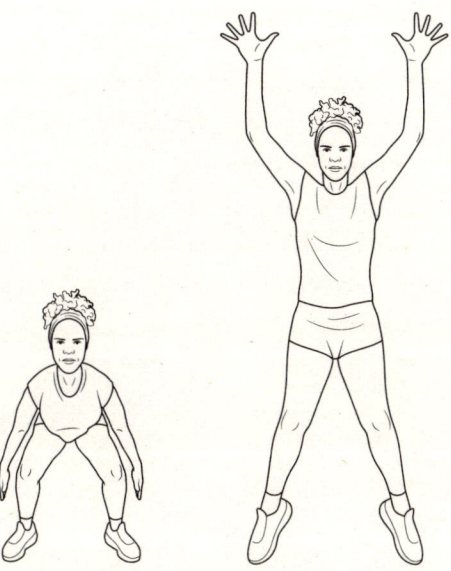

Stand with your feet shoulder-width apart, keeping your chest up and your shoulders back. Lower into a squat position, pushing your hips back as if you are about to sit in a chair. Lower your body down until you are as low as you can go. If your heels start to rise up as you lower, you have gone too far. Keep your knees aligned in the same direction as your toes. Now press through your heels and explode up into a jump. Swing your arms overhead as you jump upwards – not forwards – to get even more momentum. When coming back down, try to land softly on the balls of your feet, then settle back into your heels and bend your knees ever so slightly to absorb the impact and help you balance. As quickly as you can, lower yourself back into the squat position ready to jump up again. Repeat for the desired number of repetitions.

## SPEED SKATER

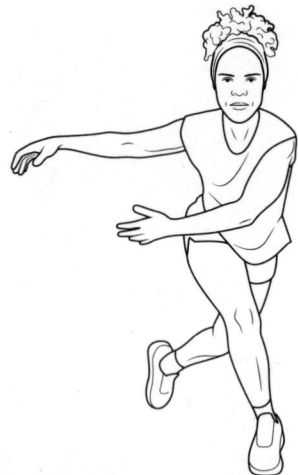

Stand with your feet shoulder-width apart, slightly bend your knees and hinge forwards at the hips. Keep your chest up and core engaged. Push off with your right leg, jumping laterally to your left and onto your left foot, and allow your right foot to trail behind you. To return, immediately push off your left leg, jumping laterally to the right. Trail the left foot behind. Keep jumping side to side for the desired number of repetitions. Get your arms involved to help propel you further to the side and control momentum – swing them in the direction you are jumping. Keep the movement controlled and fluid.

## FORWARD JUMP

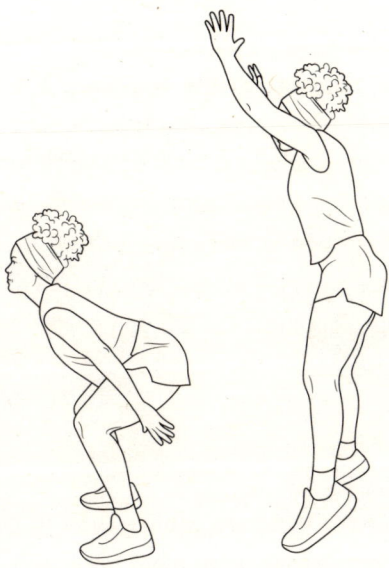

Start with your feet shoulder-width apart, engage your core and keep your chest up. Bend your knees and lower your hips *slightly*, as if preparing for a squat. Swing your arms back to start to generate momentum and then jump upwards and forwards, using your legs and arms to propel yourself (as you jump, your arms will come forwards and up above your head – think of long jump). Your aim is to jump forwards as far as is possible while being in control. You should aim to land softly on your feet, allowing your heels to drop down gently. Bend your knees to absorb impact and maintain balance. Go back to where you started and repeat for the desired number of repetitions.

> **I LOVE TO SKIP!**
>
> 'I started skipping with a rope in the pandemic as a way to keep active. It was available, easily accessible and really effective in terms of cardiovascular exercise. In the beginning I didn't think about how it would benefit my running. It was a couple of years ago that I realised that my skipping was a form of plyometric exercise. When I am running, I am thinking about my cadence, which, in terms of rhythm, is very much akin to my skipping. Often, if I'm tired in a run I will visualise myself skipping along the road. It's also been great for calf strengthening. Skipping is the gift that keeps on giving!'

## The routines

So, now you know what the moves are it's time to do them. Remember, this is not supposed to take over your life. This is about finding some time to practise some exercises that will not only support you in running but will make you feel stronger in all areas of your life – not just physical, but mental too.

Now, if all you can manage is one 20-minute session per week then I would recommend you start with the lower body session. Why? Because it will target those primary muscles that are used for running and address areas where, often, women runners report they feel niggles.

If you can manage two 20-minute sessions a week, then incorporate a core session. Three sessions? Add upper body. And for four sessions, add in plyometrics too.

This is up to you. There are no hard-and-fast rules as to how quickly you should progress, how much weight – in addition to your bodyweight – you should lift. As I have said previously, it's about how you feel. If the exercise feels too easy, how can you progress it? If the weight is too light, what else at home can you use?

The sessions

### Lower body

| Name | Reps | Sets | Rest period* |
|---|---|---|---|
| Squat | 10 | 3 | 30–60 seconds |
| Split squat | 10 each side | 3 | 30–60 seconds |
| Slouch | 5 each side | 2–3 | 30–60 seconds |

### Upper body

| Name | Reps | Sets | Rest period |
|---|---|---|---|
| Modified push-up | 5–10 | 3 | 30–60 seconds |
| Standing dumbbell arm swing | 10 each side (20 in total) | 3 | 30–60 seconds |
| Single-arm dumbbell row | 10 each side (20 in total) | 3 | 30–60 seconds |

### Core

| Name | Reps | Sets | Rest period |
|---|---|---|---|
| Half plank | Hold for up to 20 seconds | 3 | 30–60 seconds |
| Dead bug | 10 each side (20 in total) | 3 | 30–60 seconds |
| Oblique twist | 10 each side (20 in total) | 3 | 30–60 seconds |

### Plyometric

| Name | Reps | Sets | Rest period |
|---|---|---|---|
| Jump squat | 10 | 3 | 30–60 seconds |
| Speed skater | 10 each side (20 in total) | 3 | 30–60 seconds |
| Forward jump | 10 | 3 | 30–60 seconds |

*Rest for 30–60 seconds between each set of reps. For example:
**Set 1:** Perform 10 x squats and then rest for 30–60 seconds.

**Set 2:** Perform 10 x squats and then rest for 30–60 seconds.
**Set 3:** Perform 10 x squats and then rest for 30–60 seconds.

If you feel a twinge or something doesn't feel quite right? Stop and enlist some expert support.

## Common running niggles experienced by women

If there is one thing that stops women completing their journey to learn to run, it's niggles. In my experience it's not a woman's lack of motivation – because that endorphin rush is addictive – it's about her dealing with common issues that start small and seem insignificant but, when not addressed, turn into big problems that stop her running.

According to Ed, the main injuries that he sees in new runners are tendon issues: 'Your tendons are located all over your body, wherever a muscle attaches to a bone. They are strong, fibrous connective tissues and play a crucial role in facilitating movement and transmitting the force generated by your muscle contractions to your bones. They don't like change and need to be *gently* encouraged to deal with more load. Because of a lack of understanding as to what *gentle progressive load* looks like, a lot of new runners can experience tendon issues, which, if ignored, have the potential to become a stubborn and limiting pain.'

If you feel you are experiencing tendon issues and it is impacting your ability to run, seek expert help by consulting a registered physiotherapist.

Whether it's run training or strength training there are a set of principles that any runner – no matter whether you are a beginner or advanced – needs to abide by:

- Sow it (progression) – Start small and slowly build up.
- Water it (rest) – Have a break from the exercise.
- Watch it bloom (adaptation) – Your body gets stronger and adapts to what you are doing with it.

I know lots of women I have worked with over the years who get excited about running and do not take enough rest. They want to do more, they feel good, they are excited about this new form of exercise. This puppy dog syndrome can lead to too much progressive overload (aka doing too much, too soon) on the body, which, if not managed, can lead to injury.

Your body needs to be encouraged, in a way that is right for you, to tolerate more 'load' (meaning so that it can do more). Depending on your current lifestyle, learning to run is going to impose a significantly higher impact on your body, and be more physically demanding, than what you have been used to doing day to day. The golden rule is to do what you can to ensure you are in a position where your system, your beautiful body, is tolerant to that load. The way to do that is to train it – with a mixture of running and strength and conditioning – to increase its resilience and capacity.

That's what this book is here to help you do.

Common areas where you might feel niggles:

- Achilles tendon (back of the ankle) (runs from the bottom of the calf muscles to the heel bone)
- Perineal tendon (outside of the ankle)
- Tibialis posterior (inside of the ankle)
- Patella tendon (bottom of the kneecap to the top of the shin)
- Hamstring tendon (back of the thigh)

Ed says: 'Some tendon issues that runners experience can be due to foot position and mobility. Or it can be an issue emanating from the shoes they are wearing. But what I urge people to remember is that we are the *sum of all of our parts*. By this, what I mean is that your history is super important.

'What good physiotherapists are adept at doing is understanding that the niggles runners experience, more often than not, come from historical biomechanical (how your body is set up) issues. Running can bring these issues to the fore due to the force and load that is being experienced in the here and now.

'If I had a runner who came to me with a tendon issue, what I would be really interested in was of course how it started, but I'd also want to know what has happened to them historically and, as a timeline, I mean since the year dot.

'We are a product of our journey, meaning that every situation that we have found ourselves in, how we move daily, injuries we had years ago, childbirth – absolutely everything – has an impact on how you as a woman move and how your body adapts to that movement.'

## Remember – it's all connected!

'Runners come to me,' says Ed, 'who have been told that the niggles they are experiencing are due to their glutes (bum muscles) not firing (working).' It's rubbish. If your bum muscles didn't work, you wouldn't be able to stand up! However, there can often be issues in *how* the glutes are working, and especially when we see how they work in conjunction with the hamstrings and calves, which is how we need them to function when we run, as a unit.

'Often what we'll find is that the glutes are having to do too much because one of the other muscles isn't doing enough – or maybe one side is working more effectively than the other – and the clue as to why is usually in that person's history. If there is a deficit in how your muscles are able to deal with force, running will often expose this, but pain can often occur in a different area to where the actual issue is. This is why it is so important when you are seeing a physio about an issue that they are getting to the root cause of the problem rather than simply treating the symptoms.'

# The impact of childbirth on new female runners

Dr Stacy Sims, a respected sports scientist, coined the phrase 'women are not small men'. Why? Because to date – as I outlined on p. 78 – many sports and exercise science studies, and advice emanating from those studies, have been based on men. And the advice that is given to us is based on the calculation of us being 'small men'.

But we are not small men. And one of many things that we can do that men cannot do is grow and deliver children. Our pelvises are different to those of men: they are wider, as in how they sit in relation to the rest of our lower body, which is referred to as Q Angle, meaning the angle of the hip down to the knee and the knee to the ankle.

Going through pregnancy and labour is hugely traumatic for the body and it has a massive impact in terms of abdominal strength, due to our muscles being lengthened and, if we have had caesarean sections, our abdominal muscles being cut. It takes time, and patience on a woman's part, for those muscles to tighten up and do their job again. If, as women, we don't have the ability to use abdominal strength to stabilise our bodies at our hips and pelvis, this can lead to us shifting from side to side rather than moving in a forward direction while running. This can then result in issues with the lower back and iliotibial band (ITB), which give us pain on the outside of the hip and knee.

## The pelvic floor

We also need to talk about the pelvic floor. This is a group of muscles, ligaments and connective tissues located at the base of your pelvis. Think of it like a supportive hammock or sling that stretches across the bottom of your pelvis. It does a *lot* of work, and it needs you to remember to care for it!

Your pelvic floor may have taken a battering through pregnancy, got damaged during childbirth or been affected by menopause. Physical stresses and hormonal changes associated with these life events can lead to pelvic floor weakness and you may experience a host of different issues due to this.

During longer runs, I experience urine leakage even when my bladder does not feel full. I'll admit that, after pregnancy and childbirth, I didn't pay enough attention to pelvic floor exercises that were prescribed to me. If involuntary leakage is something you are worried about then I'd advise wearing a sanitary pad or period pants during your run.

Pelvic floor exercises – often referred to as Kegel exercises – can help to strengthen a woman's pelvic floor, and the great thing about them is that they can be done anywhere, at any time, and no one need know about it. I do mine while brushing my teeth; other women do theirs while waiting for the kettle to boil. Find what works for you.

### TRY IT NOW: POWER UP YOUR PELVIC FLOOR

- **Identify the right muscles** – To find your pelvic floor muscles, try stopping urination midstream. The muscles you use to do this are your pelvic floor muscles. This is purely for identification, so you can feel where your pelvic floor muscles are – it's not the exercise itself!
- **Get comfortable** – You can do this exercise lying down, sitting or standing. Find a comfortable position.
- **Contract the muscles** – Tighten your pelvic floor muscles and hold the contraction. Imagine you're trying to lift the pelvic floor upwards.
- **Hold** – Aim to hold the contraction for about three to five seconds.
- **Relax** – Release the contraction and relax for the same amount of time.
- **Repetitions** – Start with 10 repetitions and gradually work your way up to 15–20. Aim for three sets a day.

When it comes to pelvic floor strength, other than classic Kegel-type exercises, such as the one explained above, any exercise that has a glute (bum) focus will help to support your pelvic floor. In particular, exercises that involve hip rotation, too. One to try alongside the above exercise is called a hip airplane.

# HIP AIRPLANE

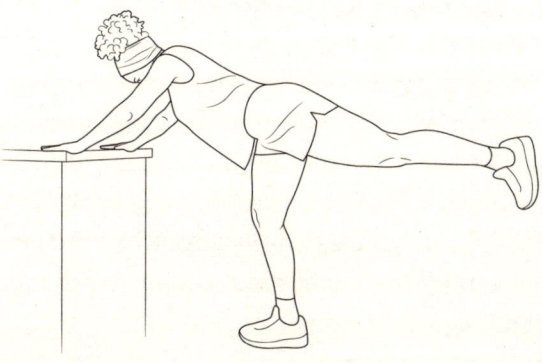

First, find something that will help to stabilise you that is about hip height – a table would work. Face the table and place your hands on it with your arms outstretched (for balance). Now stand on your right leg, ensuring you keep a slight bend at the knee, and hinge forwards at your hips so that your upper body leans forwards and your left leg extends behind you (like a T-shape) with your toes pointing down. There should be a slight bend in that left leg that is now airborne. Keep your abdominal muscles switched on (tight).

To start the exercise your hips should be facing the ground. When you're ready, slowly rotate your chest and hips open to the left side (the side of your lifted leg) so that your toes on that leg turn out to about 90 degrees and your pelvis is opening up to that left side. Remember, you are aiming to use your hip rotation and your glutes to subtly change into this position. Take it slowly and keep your balance. Go as far as is comfortable without twisting your knee or arching your back. Now rotate your hips closed by turning your torso towards your standing leg. Don't drop that back leg! The aim is to feel the muscles in your hips and glutes working to control the rotation movement outwards and inwards. Repeat this three to five times standing on the right leg and then switch position and repeat standing on the left leg.

## Your support network

I've spent years running long distances and have had to deal with a few niggles, so I'm good at leaning on sports therapists and physiotherapists when I need to. My advice to you is this: if you are pain free and can commit to doing at least one 20-minute strength and conditioning session a week it's OK to start on your 10-week learn-to-run programme. But if you have any concerns, maybe you have an ankle that has been feeling a bit stiff or your hip feels a bit strange when you have been sitting down for too long, then you might want to book to see a physiotherapist for a bit of an MOT before starting.

To find a good physiotherapist, contact your local clinic, or do some research online, and ask for the details of staff who have specialisms in sport and, if possible, specifically running. It's so important to find someone you trust, someone who has worked with other women like you. Rapport is important, so if you can arrange a 15-minute chat with them, and you like what you hear, they might just be the support that you need to help you to be able to run stronger, for longer.

CHAPTER 12

# You get out what you put in

You'll often hear runners talking about 'fuelling'. They're not referring to filling their cars with petrol, diesel or topping up the electric power charge. No, this is all about food and drink.

You'll hear them discussing what they can 'take on board' – and by that they mean chew and swallow (I know, right, why not just speak plain English?). This fuel will give them the energy to be prepared for, to complete and to recover from their run.

I had absolutely no idea what any of these terms meant before I started running and I have had so many questions from women I coach about fuelling and hydration (by that they mean drinks!).

Common questions:

- 'How long before I go on a run do I need to eat?'
- 'What types of food do I need to eat?'
- 'Does the type of food I eat depend on how much I weigh?'
- 'How many calories should those foods consist of?'
- 'Should I run with food and drink on me?'
- 'How should I carry it?'
- 'How much food and drink should I take on a run?'
- 'I've heard that fasted training is good for women. Should I not eat before I run?'

- 'But I want to lose weight and am looking to running to help me do that, so surely, eating defeats the object?'
- 'What is sports nutrition and should I use it?'

I am a running coach and a personal trainer. I am not a sports dietician. Elements of my qualifications touched, and they were light touches, on nutrition but it is not an area in which I am an expert. Thankfully there are many respected experts out there – one of whom I have asked to help write this chapter.

Renee McGregor, who we met briefly in chapter 9, is a leading sports dietitian who specialises in working with women just like you (female elite athletes!) to educate and support them on how to nurture their bodies using food and drink. How to use simple fuelling strategies to support their running performance before, during and after their runs.

And, yes, it matters for you as a beginner. So, let's get into it.

## Me and food

You'll know from chapter 1 that I started running for mental illness reasons. To reclaim some sense of identity. To be a better mum. And, over days, weeks and months I did indeed get that. Running became my go-to. You'll also remember that in that chapter I talked about being 32kg (5 stone) overweight post-partum, about being worried about my big, milky boobs hitting me in the face if I ran, about finding clothing to jog in that covered all of my wobbly bits that at that time I felt I wanted to hide.

I always had a complicated relationship with food. Therapy has helped me realise much of this battle comes from growing up in a single-parent family, on the breadline, being in receipt of food bank parcels – before food banks were ever a thing – and therefore always feeling fear around the scarcity of food. My mum always told me and my sister to 'clean the plates', so that's what we did – we licked the plates clean.

I love food. I always have and, as a kid, I was stocky. Not overweight, but stocky. I became pregnant at 17 and had my first baby at 18. What I loved about being pregnant was not feeling as if I had to restrict my food. I was growing a human being, so if I wanted something to eat then it wasn't really me wanting it, it was the baby! This led to weight gain during my pregnancies and, for years, a cycle of yo-yo dieting was my norm. As part of that yo-yo dieting I would use exercise (aerobics classes mainly) as a way to punish myself if I had a bad day. Or to go deeper into calorie restriction if I had a good day.

But why am I sharing this with you? Because I *know* that there will be a proportion of you women reading this book who will have done the same – who do the same. That you too may have had, or have, a complicated relationship with food. Some of you will have even picked up this book because someone told you – or worse, you have read – that of all the activities you can do, running is the one that burns the most calories in an hour. Maybe you have a friend, a family member or you follow someone online who has transformed their bodies, and they put all of this down to running.

Running is so good for you and it's not only because of the amount of calories that you might burn while doing it. It's about the magnitude of other benefits that it gives you from a mental, physical and social perspective. A side effect of running is that – yes – you might lose weight and gain muscle tone, but that really is a side effect. I know women who run and don't lose weight at all because they don't do it for that. But what they gain is confidence, fitness and a pride in 'seeing what their body can do'. They eat to run, not run to eat.

# What is fuel?

It doesn't matter how fast you run, whether you walk/run – and if you choose to follow my 5K plan you *will* be walking as well as running – or what time of the day you run. You need to ensure your body has enough fuel to perform.

You need to eat and drink.

You need to ensure you have enough carbohydrates in your system to enable your body to do what it needs to – no matter 'what' that performance looks like. If your body does not have enough carbohydrate to feed your body, and your brain, the energy it needs to move forwards, you will not feel joy in this process. If it does not have enough carbohydrate, you may even feel unwell during the process. If it does not have enough carbohydrate, you may not achieve the goal that you have set yourself.

You do not have to eat all of the time but get into the habit of eating a portion of carbohydrate as part of your breakfast, a portion of carbohydrate as part of your lunch and a portion of carbohydrate as part of your evening meal.

## What does a portion of carbohydrate look like?

Look at your hand. Now make a fist. That fist size that you have made is the approximate size of the portion of carbohydrate that it is advised we eat at every meal.

I admit, I often go above a 'fist' portion, because a) I like food and b) I love carbs. Some examples of the foods that I include in my pre-run carbohydrate loading include:

- A bowl of porridge with honey and nuts
- Two slices of toast with peanut butter
- A medium-sized jacket potato with cheese and beans or cottage cheese
- A banana (use your imagination and pretend you've scrunched up the banana into a fist)
- A bagel with butter and jam
- Two slices of buttered malt loaf (my number one go-to running food)
- A large bread roll with cheese and pickle
- One or one and a half squished-up Snickers bars

There are times when life is really testing, and time is not my friend. So, yes, sometimes lunch does look like a bagel with melted butter topped with a banana. Sometimes it looks like two slices of malt loaf and a packet of salt and vinegar crisps. Sometimes it's a Snickers bar, the 'Red Ambulance' (runners' speak for full-fat Coca-Cola) and the promise to have more nutritional balance tomorrow.

But one thing I do know is that if I go into a run practice session and I do not have enough carbohydrates flowing around my body, I feel awful. I feel weak. I feel sick. I feel disappointed in myself. And the reason for all these feelings and so many more is because my body does not have enough fast-release carbohydrate (glucose) – which is the preferred energy source used by the body – to enable the biological processes that need to take place for you to run.

Why? Because it's directing the energy that it does have to your critical biological and cognitive processes – you know, the ones keeping you alive! Your heart, your lungs, your brain.

> **FUEL IN THE TANK**
>
> 'If I know I am going out on a run, I always have porridge with banana and honey for breakfast. It's my petrol and ensures I'm going to reach my destination on the run. Whatever that distance may be!'

For your body to adapt to running efficiently, effectively and with JOY, you must feed it. *At least* three meals a day. *At least* a fistful of carbohydrate at each meal.

If you really want to start and, most importantly, stay running, you must fuel your body. I urge you to eat food that will help your body, and mind, perform during each running session I have designed for you. And it's about more than five portions of fruit and vegetables a day – or whatever the current public health messaging is at the moment. It's about the carbohydrates pre run and protein post run. It's about the time window you allow yourself to eat before and after a run to avoid tummy issues and ensure you are feeding your body what it needs to repair.

I so badly want you to eat to enjoy your running journey and – believe me when I say – restricting your diet when learning to run isn't the path of joy. So, let's get some premium fuel into you so you can reap the rewards when you are out there running.

> **NOURISH YOUR BODY**
>
> 'I've never done restrictive dieting because I believe I have to have a strong and capable body. To have that I need to fuel it correctly. Rather than depriving myself, I focus on foods that nourish my body and support my running and overall well-being. This approach has helped me maintain the energy and strength I need for my runs, while also supporting me to have a healthy, sustainable relationship with food.'

## When should I fuel?

This is about figuring out what works for you and, as you go on this journey, your experimentation and the positive (and negative!) experiences that you have that will inform your eating patterns. But – as a rule of thumb – the advice is to eat anywhere between one and three hours before you run. I know, that's quite the time frame and that's why I want to reinforce the importance of finding what works for you.

I have trained myself to be able to eat 30–60 minutes before I go on a run. I do this because, in the past, I have struggled with unexplained blood sugar highs and lows, which, when experiencing lows on a run, have knocked me for six. Due to this, I decided to start training my gut to get comfortable with digesting carbohydrate-rich food close to when I start running. This strategy absolutely doesn't work for everyone; it's taken me years to perfect and I know what foods work well for me. For you as new runners, I'd advise the one-to three-hour window.

I do well with breakfast-type snacks that are solid in nature, such as toast, a bagel or malt loaf. I don't do well with foods that swish around in my tummy, such as milky cereal or shakes. You may be different.

If I am going to run at lunchtime (otherwise known as doing a Runch!) and the window is more than three hours since breakfast, then I will fuel 30–60 minutes before on a snack like a banana or a piece of malt loaf. That is sufficient to keep me fuelled (if I have eaten breakfast) for up to an hour of running.

# Recovery fuelling – helping your body to heal

As well as fuelling to prepare your body to perform, it's important not to forget about what you consume post run to fuel your body's ability to *recover*.

Every time you run, biological adaptions are happening. These are part of making you a stronger runner. A by-product of your running practice is that your muscles will experience micro-tears that are a normal part of the process. If you've ever experienced DOMS (delayed onset muscle soreness) then you'll know how this feels – but it's a good sign and part of the process of your body being put under strain and adapting. Amino acids are responsible for the muscular build, and repair. Protein contains amino acids, which is why consuming protein as part of your post-run recovery meal or snack is *so* important. As part of every meal it's important, but definitely as part of your post-run fuelling. If you do not have enough protein in your diet from real food or sports nutrition, your body will not adapt to the running practice you are doing, and you may also be more prone to running-related injury. This is even more important as you get older and especially when you are in perimenopause and menopause.

So, your post-run meal should really look like a mixture of carbohydrates (to replenish energy stores) *and* protein (to repair muscle).

Renee's top five recovery meals:

- Eggs on toast
- Chicken salad wrap
- Chickpea soup and a roll
- Sports recovery shake made with milk, added oats and a banana
- Baked potato with tuna

As Renee talks about in her amazing book, which I urge you to go and buy, *Fuel For Thought*, food doesn't have to be complicated. It is not rocket science. Fuelling for running performance – let's call it running joy – is about choosing food and drinks that are specific to *your* needs.

You are unique and what works for me, or a friend that you know who runs, or someone you follow online, might not work for you. When it comes to fuelling, the fun – as someone who *loves* finding new sources of carbohydrates and protein – is in the experimenting!

## Do I need to take food and drink out while I am running?

The scientists will tell you no. The coach in me says, 'It's up to you.' Many of the beginners I have coached turn up to that first session clutching a bottle of water as if their life depended on it. They don't know what to expect. What they *do* know is that they are going to be exercising a little more intensively than they have been used to. So, who am I to tell them that they can't carry a bottle of water?!

I am here to empower you to make decisions about the way that *you* want to incorporate running into your life. And if that means carrying a bottle of water while you run, then so be it. I have no idea how much water you have drunk today. I don't know at what rate you start to sweat. I don't know whether you would be classed as a 'salty sweater' so, because of these unknowns, it's important to do what feels right to you.

> **ARE YOU A SALTY SWEATER?!**
>
> We all sweat at different rates and the levels of sodium (salt) included in our sweat differ. One of the simplest ways to tell if you are a salty sweater is to look for white marks on your clothes, headband or hat post run (salty sweat tends to dry white). Some people see white marks on their skin. Some people can *taste* their salty sweat. FYI I am not a salty sweater, but I have friends who are and it just means that they may need to take on more electrolytes (*see* p.207) pre, during and post run than I do.

The same applies to food. If you have had a carbohydrate-rich breakfast, lunch or dinner pre run then you should be adequately fuelled to be able to do the run session that I have prescribed for you without taking anything to eat out with you.

And I really do want to encourage you to get into that habit of eating three balanced meals – consisting of protein, carbohydrates and fats – a day.

You will find that, after a few of my sessions, your confidence in what you need to eat and drink pre, during and post run will start to build. Often, I find that the women who start out clutching water bottles do then leave them at home, or in the car, from week three onwards.

My sessions are designed to last no longer than an hour maximum (and that's in the latter stages of the plan). If you have fuelled your body adequately and have hydrated yourself so you do not feel thirsty then you should be absolutely fine.

### THE SCIENCE BIT

Science shows that our bodies have enough stored energy to keep moving well for up to 90 minutes. If you are out for longer than 90 minutes, then that's when your energy stores will start to get low and you will need to refuel on the go.

You're not likely to be out longer than 60 minutes on any of the runs I have created for you. However, if for any reason you haven't fuelled well in the days leading up to your run, or on the day of the run itself, then that's different. That's when I would advocate having a little 'scooby snack' – something that you can have on you 'just in case'. A snack that that can release carbohydrate into your system fast.

Good scooby snacks for runners include:

- Flapjack
- Snickers bar

- Dextrose tablets
- A malt loaf bar
- A jam sandwich
- Jelly babies
- Sports gel
- Sports beans (basically jelly beans)

## Keeping it real?

I can't write a chapter on nutrition and ignore the sports nutrition market – a market that has been created to cater to the demands of athletes of all abilities. A market that is estimated to be worth $94 billion by 2033.

So, what is sports nutrition? Why does it matter and what, as a new runner, can it do for you? Well, when you hear about sports nutrition for runners, people will mainly be referring to the following products in particular:

**Sports gels** – A small pouch, normally no bigger than the palm of your hand, containing a gel-like substance (sounds appealing, doesn't it?). The gel has been formulated to give you energy that can be consumed (sucked) easily while on the move. The make-up of the recipe, normally containing between 25g (1oz) and 60g (2.5oz) of carbohydrate, can be absorbed by your body quickly, delivering the energy you need to fuel your run.

**Sports bars** – A drier bar that can contain a multitude of ingredients that act in the same way as those in a sports gel but are slower-release. This is normally a dense product and, once again, will deliver a set amount of carbohydrate, protein and other nutrients. You'd normally consume these bars pre run or, for longer distances, as part of a wider fuelling strategy. I often use these as pre-run snacks if I don't have time to eat a more balanced real meal.

**Sports drinks** – Drinks that have been formatted – think Lucozade – to deliver a mix of carbohydrate and other essential nutrients (plus electrolytes) to be consumed pre, during and/or post run.

**Protein shakes** – These come in either powder or ready-to-drink form. Powders can normally be mixed with water or milk to create a 300–400ml (10–13.5fl oz) drink and, on average, can deliver up to 25g (1oz) of protein per serving. If made with milk, these are a great recovery choice after a harder or longer run.

> Are you a lover of cow's milk? If so, read on! Studies have shown that cow's milk provides benefits for muscle repair AND may also help to prevent DOMS (Delayed Onset Muscle Soreness). Milk offers a great mix of protein, carbohydrate and electrolytes that support muscle recovery and hydration. The combination of these things also makes it a really great rehydration drink. So, whether as a stand-alone drink, or mixed with protein power (as above) milk is wonder fuel.

Many of the runners who I coach, both brand new and those who have been running for years, love chocolate milk as their source of protein. Not only does it taste great, but it delivers a perfect ratio of carbs to protein (3:1) for recovery post run. It's also very reasonably priced.

Sports nutrition has its place. Our lives can be busy and, sometimes, with the best will in the world, the convenience of a pre-made gel, bar or drink is what we need in order to ensure we prepare for and recover from our runs and are ready to take on whatever else life has to throw at us.

There are a whole host of different products out there; there will be some that you love and some that you hate. In the many years that I have been running I have tested lots. Some I loved to begin with and – due to overconsumption – grew tired of very quickly. Some made me feel nauseous and tasted of bland goo.

If there was one sports nutrition product that I rely on above all else, it's my protein powder shake or chocolate milk. No matter what age you are, protein matters. It's absolutely essential for recovery. A tip that I'd give you is to prepare it before you go on your run. It's normally one scoop of protein powder to 250–300ml (8.5–10fl oz) of water. Once mixed, put it in the fridge and then, when you come home, it's easily quaffable and tastes (almost) like a McDonald's milkshake. On average a good protein shake will deliver 20–25g (around 1oz) of protein per serving, which will help you towards your recommended daily protein goal.

> On average, you should be looking to consume 1.2–2 grams of protein per kilogram of bodyweight per day. Please see p. 150 for information on protein requirements for perimenopausal women as they are slightly higher.

## Keeping hydrated

Do you know how much water we as women are supposed to consume a day? Well, for the average woman (hey, who are you calling average?!) it's 6–8 cups or glasses a day. But remember, as with any standard nutritional advice, you are not an average woman. You are a runner! And, as a new runner, that number doesn't really apply to you because – as I have said before – due to the increase in consistent activity you may need more.

No matter how far or how fast you run, hydrating your body is important. Please don't wait to sweat to give yourself permission to take on board water and, if you are already thirsty, then that's a sign that you may already be dehydrated. As for nutrition, it's important to think about what you are drinking pre and post run.

I am a woman of a certain age. I get hot (and sweat) just going about my business. I sweat at work. I sweat walking the dog and playing with the grandkids. I sweat in bed at night. All of this means I am losing essential salts from my body. It means we – you and me – may have a mineral balance that is off kilter and, therefore, just drinking water isn't going to alleviate the symptoms that are associated with being dehydrated.

Possible signs and symptoms of dehydration (not exhaustive) are:

- Dark-coloured urine (it should be pale straw in colour)
- Tiredness

- GI issues (see below)
- Sensation of heavy legs (even at the beginning of a run)
- Nausea
- Headache
- Low blood pressure (dizziness)

## Electrolytes

So how can we redress that balance? Well, first, you can ensure that you are taking sips of water regularly. And by sips, I mean sips. There really is no great benefit from chugging down a litre of water at teatime because you forgot to drink during the day. You'll just find yourself on the toilet more. Remember: small sips, often.

Also think about electrolytes. Electrolytes are basically effervescent tablets or a powder that you can add to water and use to replace some of the sodium and other minerals that you have lost through sweating. Lately, and upon the advice of Renee, I have been adding electrolytes to 400ml (13.5fl oz) of water and sipping it throughout the day. (You can get all kinds of different-flavoured ones. Mine is currently watermelon.) I sip this mix even on rest days. I have to say, I feel better for it. If it is a running day, I will drink more of this mix, and if it is a hot day, I will drink even more. I listen to my body.

Easy-to-take electrolytes:

- DIY electrolyte mix – You can make this easily at home. Dilute 300ml (10fl oz) of water with 300ml (10fl oz) of fruit juice and ¼ tsp of salt. Voilà!
- Electrolyte capsules (taken as a tablet with water)
- Electrolyte powder or effervescent tablet (mixed with water)

# Why lighter isn't faster

When I took up running, I was carrying more weight than I would have liked. I was three months post-partum and breastfeeding. Losing weight, at that time, wasn't the main driver for taking up running. I remember thinking, 'If I lose some weight via the process, then that would be nice' but I mostly just wanted to help my postnatal depression.

Women take up running for all sorts of reasons and it would be remiss of me not to address the simple fact that many women, maybe even you, want to use it as a tool to lose weight. You might have decided to use running alongside an eating regime – of which there are many – with the aim being to eat fewer calories than you burn.

Often, if you have some body fat to lose – and are following a sensible diet – you *will* see changes, and you may even see them quite fast. But, if the energy you are taking in through food and drink is not enough to give your body what it needs to function and live and run, you will not feel good.

To put it bluntly, you will feel shit.

> **YOUR BODY NEEDS CARBS**
>
> 'When I started running, I was afraid of carbohydrates. I saw them as the enemy and definitely underfuelled. This restriction affected my mood, my performance and my recovery. I've learned that I need to fuel my body to do the things I want to do.'

If you do not give your body what it needs, because you are not taking in enough calories, you will not have the energy you need to run, or for your body to efficiently adapt to the practices that I will be encouraging.

Being lighter, in and of itself, will *not* make you a better runner. In fact, underfuelling your body as a runner can lead to serious health implications.

Renee is one of the leading experts on REDs (relative energy deficiency in sport) – when athletes don't get enough fuel to support energy demands. She also researches orthorexia – a medical condition in which the sufferer systemically avoids specific foods they believe to be harmful. Renee works tirelessly to debunk myths around the female athlete body. And one of these myths is around the topic of, 'If I am lighter, I will be faster.'

Over to Renee: 'One of the difficulties is that when anyone initially loses weight, their running does improve temporarily, and they attribute this success to their weight.

'However, while this number or body composition may have delivered once upon a time, it is not reproducible in the short, medium or longer term because the body cannot sustain this level of underfuelling without turning on compensatory behaviours that leave your body weak and at high risk of injury. Being lighter does not make you faster. Fuelling for your changing lifestyle, being consistent and being strong and healthy for you does!'

## Gut instinct

We've talked a lot about food and drink so it would be weird if I didn't talk about how your body might handle it. Who can forget, and it's easy to find online if you haven't seen it, the time when one of the UK's best female marathon runners had to pull over to the side of the road – during her race – to have a poo.

Shit happens. It's a fact of life but, for female runners, it seems so much more embarrassing, something we don't like to talk about. How your body takes in, digests, uses and gets rid of what you eat and drink is individual to you.

First, if you have less blood flow to aid digestion, and you're jiggling up and down (as you will be when running) with food in your gut, your body is going to try to get rid of that. It's a mechanical response. And also remember that, while running, oxygenated blood is being sent to other working muscles in your legs, arms, core, brain, etc., which means that there is less blood flowing to, for example, your colon. This can cause irritation and, you've guessed it, feelings of discomfort. Part of your practice of running is training your gut to get better at dealing with what's there. It's about being mindful that certain foods may cause more problems. As I've said, I avoid eating milky cereals or foods that are too wet. Stodgier foods work better for me. Foods with a high fibre content – that are designed to bind and stay in your system for longer – can also be a trigger for gut issues while running, so it might be worth reducing those foods pre run. It's the same with high-fat foods. They take longer to digest and they stick around in your gut longer, therefore making them more likely to cause gastrointestinal, or GI, distress.

Foods that may trigger tummy issues and should be avoided in the hour or two before a run are:

- Fibrous foods like broccoli, spinach, kale, brown rice, wholewheat bread or pasta.
- High-sugar foods like cakes, chocolate and white bread.
- High-fat foods like processed foods, dairy and fried foods.

Now, as you'll see above, the things that I list as my 'power carbohydrates' do fall into these categories, but they work for me and do not mess with my GI. However, I am well aware that, for some of you, they may be triggers while others will be absolutely fine. Just keep an eye on what you are eating and how it interacts with your GI and you will find what works for you, too.

### A HYDRATED GUT IS A HAPPY GUT

Renee: 'Hydration is one of the key things to think about if your stomach is upset. If you haven't got the right salt/fluid balance and are dehydrated, then that will mean you are concentrating the contents of your stomach and those contents will want to "release".'

It's also important to be mindful of how fast you are consuming foods pre run. For example, if you are in a rush and ingest, for example, a high-carbohydrate gel or piece of food quickly, then that's quite a large hit of sugar to your system, which it can find difficult to deal with.

And, if you have tummy issues that you are working through, then it's always handy to pick a route that passes by locations with toilets or, like I did, take up trail running and invest in a runner's shovel!

## SUPPLEMENTS

There is a lot of noise out there about sports supplements, especially for women. Creatine, collagen, L-glutamine, cherry juice and others are all cited as being beneficial for athletes. Whether or not they will benefit you depends on many factors, not least the type, intensity and duration of the exercise you are doing. I am not a dietitian, so I advise you to do your own research using reputable sources, such as Renee's books or Anita Bean's *The Runner's Cookbook*.

However, there are two, which I've previously mentioned, that I can safely say are beneficial:

- Vitamin D – You will likely need to increase your vitamin D. As a runner you will need it for muscular recovery. We all feel the ache in our legs from running at some point – it happens because every time we exercise, we create micro-tears in our muscles, this creates that ache and, as it disappears, that's our muscles repairing. Vitamin D helps this recovery process and eases DOMS. If DOMS last for a long time, and happen on every single run, it's a sign that you might be low in vitamin D. Keeping your levels topped up in the autumn and winter months is recommended by the NHS for everyone.
- Iron – I spoke earlier about the symptoms associated with lower iron levels (tiredness, fatigue, brain fog, etc. – *see* p. 154). Iron deficiency can have a real impact on your running. Look out for signs and consult a pharmacist or your GP if advice is needed, and take a supplement as advised.

## CHAPTER 13

# Miles and smiles

Well. Here you are. You made it to your first finish line.

You've done all the reading and, I hope, learned a lot about the physical and mental process of running but – most importantly – I hope you've learned a bit about yourself, too.

Maybe you wrote questions in the margins of this book? If so, reach out to me on social media and ask away. I will be only too happy to help or, if I can't, I will certainly guide you to a resource or some other qualified expert that can.

For you to even manage to get to this chapter shows your commitment to learning to run. And that's all I want from you right now. A commitment to try. Because, already, you have carved out – even if only 10 minutes a day – chunks of time to start to understand every element associated with this life-changing process.

You have already committed. Kudos to you!

I know you may be feeling nervous because 'this is it'. It's the stage when you are going to start to put everything you have read about in the previous pages into effect. You are going to start practising your running. You are going to be at that point I was at in 2009. Maybe feeling all of the same emotions that I did. I get it.

You may feel anxiety and fear – the 'But what if I can't do it?' sensation. Remember, you are not alone in experiencing these thoughts and feelings. Hundreds of thousands of other women do. It is totally normal. Still, to this day, when I start a new block of training or stand on a start line, I get those feelings, too. 'Can I do this?' 'Have I got time?' 'Have I done enough?' 'Am I good enough?'

Every single time, the answer is a big fat YES.

Through commitment and consistency, you can run. With the support of this book, you can run. By sharing your intention to learn to run with close friends and family, you can run. And by connecting with women, and new communities, that are out there waiting to support you, you can run.

Are you ready to start?

Let's do this.

## Frequency of practice

In the plan, I am asking you to practise your running two times per week. That's it. Honestly, that is all you need! Based on the sessions that I give you, you should be out for no longer than one hour. Now, I say this with a caveat. I cannot – and do not want to – be prescriptive about the time you are out running for. As we have discussed, you are unique and how you will feel on any given day will be different. Some days you will feel like a speed demon (remember, around ovulation time) and others you'll feel a lot slower. And that is OK. No one, and I mean no one, is judging you and if they try to, send them my way! Please aim to give yourself grace and the space to practise.

What I will say, as I have seen it many times, is to please stick to two days per week, especially in the first half of the programme. If you want to do more practice to support your running then add in more strength and conditioning sessions (you should be doing a minimum of one 20-minute session of S&C anyway). I have seen many women who, high on the endorphin rush of learning to run, start to practise three or four times a week. Why? Because they feel so damn good! But this can cause problems in terms of overtraining because the programme I have designed ensures gentle progression and adaptation to running, to get your body used to running in a way that is sustainable and, as far as possible, to negate niggles or injury. Pushing your body too far and too fast will not do you any favours. Even if you think you can handle it, please be mindful.

> **WHAT IS OVERTRAINING?**
>
> Overtraining happens when you exercise too much without adequate rest, pushing your body beyond its ability to recover. It can lead to fatigue, injuries, decreased performance and burnout.

In a perfect world, I want you to end this 10-week journey hungry for more. Because you feel great. Because you have achieved your goal of running 5K your way. Because you are niggle and injury free. Because you have found a love for running.

Remember, it's a marathon, not a sprint. (Well, not quite a marathon, yet – but who knows where this will lead!)

# The sessions

Each of the sessions in the training plan has five sections.

1. The warm-up
2. Mobility
3. The session
4. The cool-down
5. Stretching

Each section is important in its own right and my advice to you is to not skip any. They each serve a purpose, as I will explain below. Also, each feeds into, and out of, the other and as a whole ensures the session gives your body – and mind – all it needs to progress you safely through the 10-week programme.

## 1 The warm-up

Giving your body and mind time to warm up and prepare for the practice you are about to do is so important. I like to use the analogy of defrosting a car on a winter's day. You turn it on, dial up the heat and sit there – depending on the age of the car you have – until the ice on the windows melts and the inside temperature increases. In a sense, that's what we are doing when we warm up. We are prepping our bodies in the same way.

An effective warm-up involves doing all of the following:

- **Increasing blood flow** – To your muscles and joints and making them more flexible, thus reducing the risk of strains or injuries. Your joints will also be lubricated, which will help them move more efficiently.
- **Increasing heart rate** – You need to prepare your heart for what is coming up by gently allowing your heart rate to increase in preparation for a little more intense activity.
- **Ensuring you'll move better** – When your muscles are warmer, they will contract and relax much more effectively, and this will make you a better-co-ordinated and more efficient runner.
- **Reducing the risk of injury** – Cold muscles are more prone to tears and strains. Spending some time warming up will help prevent these.
- **Getting you in the zone** – Your warm-up will help you transition from rest to play. To focus on yourself and the run practice ahead of you.

Please do not skip your warm-up. You'll see that even five minutes is enough to start to get your body and mind prepared.

## 2 Mobility

Mobility is an important next step in the warm-up process. Incorporating some mobility exercises will help your joints to move a little more freely through their full range of motion, which will reduce stiffness and discomfort. I want you to have freely moving hips, knees and ankles, etc., which will help you to run better.

From head to toe – here are some exercises that will help:

## NECK ROTATIONS (SIDE TO SIDE)

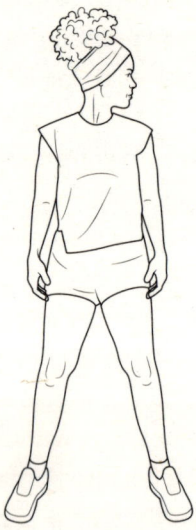

Stand tall, core engaged, with your arms hanging at the sides of your body. Do not place your hands on your hips (keep the shoulders relaxed). Keep the gaze forwards while slowly turning your head to the right. The aim is to align your chin with your shoulder. Hold for 2–3 seconds and then slowly turn to the left. Repeat this about 8–10 times per side. This exercise will improve rotation and reduce stiffness and tension in the neck and upper spine.

## NECK TILTS (FORWARDS AND BACKWARDS)

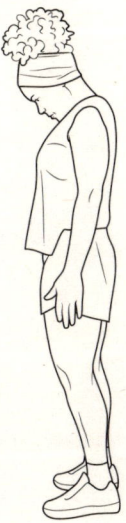

Stand tall, core engaged, with your arms hanging at the sides of your body. Do not place your hands on your hips (keep the shoulders relaxed). Slowly lower your chin to your chest, feeling a slight stretch in the back of your neck. Hold it for 3–5 seconds and then slowly tilt your head back (looking up). Hold for 3–5 seconds and then return to centre. Repeat 8–10 times. This exercise will relieve any tension in the neck and improve its range of motion.

## ARM CIRCLES

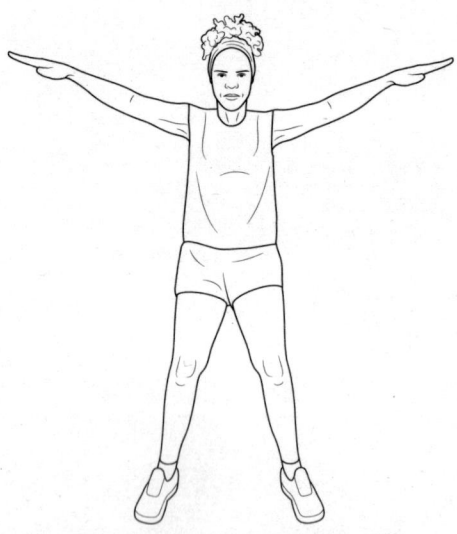

Stand tall, core engaged, with your feet shoulder-width apart. Now extend your arms out straight to the sides of your body at shoulder height (forming a T-shape). Start off by making small circles forwards with your arms, gradually increasing to larger circles. After about 10–15 seconds, reverse the direction of the circle (backward circles) for the same amount of time. This exercise will loosen up your shoulders, improve your range of motion and improve your posture and arm movement.

## STANDING HIP CIRCLES

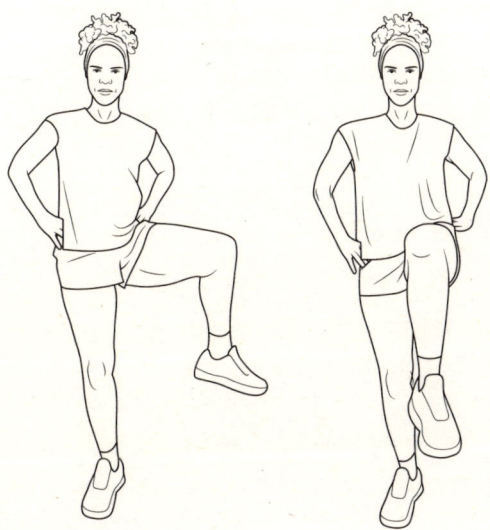

Stand tall (use a wall for support if you need to), with your core engaged and lift one knee to hip height. Rotate your knee outwards in a big circle and then bring it back inwards (continuing that circular motion) to the starting position. Repeat 8–10 times per leg. This exercise will improve your hip range and motion.

## SQUAT

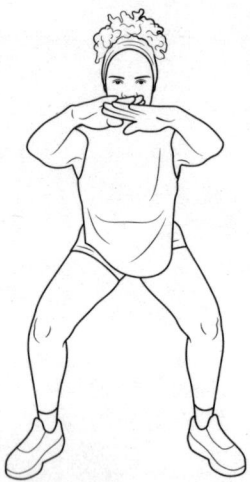

Stand with your feet shoulder-width apart with your core engaged and your toes slightly pointing out (think about them pointing towards the 11 and 1 o'clock marks on a clock). Push your bum as if to lower yourself to sit down, keeping your chest as high as you can and clasping your hands in front of you. Once you feel your heels start to rise, bring yourself back up to standing position. Inhale on the way down and exhale on the way up. Repeat 10–15 times. This exercise will improve hip, ankle and knee mobility.

## ANKLE ROTATIONS

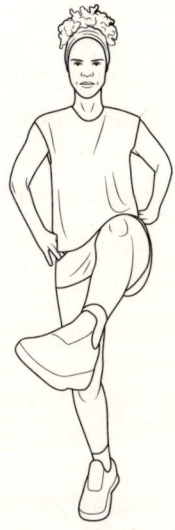

Stand tall, keeping your core engaged and chest high. Lift one foot off the ground (using a wall for support if you need to). Roll your ankle in circular motions 10 times in each direction. Once done, repeat on the other ankle. This exercise increases ankle mobility, reducing the risk of sprains.

## 3 The sessions

The plan that I have designed for you takes inspiration from a host of running plans that I have followed, loved using and redesigned for my own runners. It includes sessions that will breed consistency while also, I hope, being fun. These have been designed to bring variety to your run practice and allow you to really feel what your body is telling you on that day. It is based on gentle progression, which allows your body to adapt to the stimulus (terrain, ups, downs, flats, effort pace, etc.) placed on it.

### Remember, RPE?!

We've covered a lot of miles since we talked about rate of perceived exertion (RPE), so here is a reminder.

### Rate of perceived exertion

| RPE scale | Effort level | Activity |
| --- | --- | --- |
| 0 | Rest | |
| 1 | Really easy | This might look like a walk. Breathing will be very light. You could sing if you wanted to. |
| 2 | Easy | This might look like a brisk walk, gentle run/walk or slow jog. You can talk in complete sentences. Breathing will be light. |
| 3 | Moderate | You are breathing a bit deeper. This would be a pace you could hold consistently for the required time. You can still hold a conversation, but sentences might be shorter. |
| 4 | Sort of hard | This might look like a longer period, or a slightly faster period, of running. It will feel a bit harder. You will breathe even deeper. It's comfortably uncomfortable. |
| 5 | Hard | This might look like a session where I ask you to run intervals or hill repeats. You are going to be working hard. You will only be able to utter a few words. |
| 6 | Hard + | You will be breathing even harder. Fewer words being uttered. |

| 7 | Really hard | Your breathing is deep and laboured. You will only be able to run for shorter bursts. |
|---|---|---|
| 8 | Really hard + | Very deep and very laboured breathing. No words. |
| 9 | Really, really hard | You will be giving it all you can. |
| 10 | Maximal | Maximum effort. |

For some women it makes it easier to think about a traffic-light system:

- Amber: RPE levels 1–2
- Green: RPE levels 3–4
- Red: RPE levels 5–10

Please remember, how you 'feel' will change regularly based on all of the contributing factors we have discussed previously. If a walk with purpose feels like RPE 4 (green) and I have asked you to work at RPE 4, then guess what? Walk! Only you know how you are feeling on any given day. My main priority is breeding consistency in you, so move in a way that *feels* right for you. Just keep moving.

## The sessions explained

**Walk with purpose** – You are walking with purpose. Purpose means you are standing tall, chest open, shoulders back. Your arms are swinging, with elbows bent between 45 and 90 degrees, intentionally at your sides. Imagine there is someone, or something, ahead of you that you would really like to get to. You are on a mission to get to them. But you are *not* running. Some might call this a 'brisk' walk.

**Run to feel** – This run is very much about dialling into those different RPE levels – listening into your body and responding to the cues that you are receiving. Normally these runs will be at RPE 3–4 (conversational, forever pace).

**Out and back** – These routes serve as good 'Where am I now?' runs (if you want them to). For example, if you complete an out-and-back run at the start of the programme and make a note of how far out you got in a certain amount of time, you can repeat the run further on in your programme and compare the two. I bet – if you have been consistent – you will see a marked improvement. These runs can provide a great confidence boost.

**Mounds of opportunity** – These are your hill runs, where you are going to be practising your ascending and descending. You may have a favourite hill, or a hill you would like to focus on, and if so, great. Just like the out-and-back runs, picking a specific hill to do these sessions on can be a good marker for 'where you are' as you progress through your run practice. But also, I would say go out and run different hills, too. Where there is a hill, there is an opportunity.

**Fartlek** – I know, right?! What a name. Fartlek is a Swedish word, and it means 'speed play'. On these runs you will be playing around with your effort. You might be running comfortably and then choose to run faster to, say, the next lamppost. Then you might go back to running comfortably again while thinking about where else you might speed up again. You get to pick the points.

**Effort play** – This is all about the transition from walking to comfortable running to faster running and then going back down that scale again. How does it feel to transition up and down? There is no time prescription on how long you stay at each level. That is your call. But I want you to feel that marked difference in RPE as you move up and down the RPE levels.

**Gratitude run** – Gratitude, in running and in life, is so important. These runs are about remembering – while you run – all that you are grateful for. And that needs to include yourself, too – to give yourself gratitude for the progress you are making and, through every step, reconfirming and honouring the commitment you made to yourself.

So, enough talk. Here it is.

## MY 5K AND ME

'Running to me was boring. I'd prefer to be playing squash or some other exciting sport. But a friend of mine encouraged me to try to run 5K with her. Once we got into it, what I loved were the different sessions we were instructed to do. It added a bit of excitement, and I particularly liked the Fartleks (I still giggle at the name). The mix of sessions in my 10-week training plan kept me engaged and got me to my first Parkrun. I loved it. And I've continued to run with the group I joined, staying at 5K, as that's a distance I like, since then.'

Your 10-week couch to 5K training plan

## WEEK 1

### WARM-UP
5-minute walk with purpose (RPE 2/amber) followed by mobility work.

### RUN 1

**OUT AND BACK**
Jog for 2 minutes (RPE 3/green) followed by a walk recovery (RPE 2/amber) for 2 minutes. Aim to repeat this run/walk protocol for 12 minutes.

### COOL-DOWN

**GENTLE WALK COOL-DOWN**
(RPE 1/amber) for 5 minutes followed by gentle stretching.

### RUN 2
Not this week.

### NOTES
The likelihood is that you will feel some delayed onset muscle soreness (DOMS). This is normal.

# WEEK 2

### WARM-UP
5-minute walk with purpose (RPE 2/amber) followed by mobility work.

## RUN 1

### OUT AND BACK
6-minute out-and-back run at a ratio of 2:2 (RPE 3/green:RPE 2/amber).

If you are feeling good, you can try to extend this to 7 minutes out and 7 minutes back.

## COOL-DOWN

### WALK COOL-DOWN
(RPE 1/amber) for 5 minutes followed by gentle stretching.

## RUN 2

### FARTLEK
I want you to use the 2:2 run (RPE 3/green:RPE 2/amber) protocol to go out for 15 minutes.

## NOTES

**RUN 1**
How far do you get from your house in 5 or 7 minutes by using the run/walk strategy? Make a note of it.

**RUN 2**
How do you feel? Are you tired? Are any areas of your body feeling tight? Really tune into your body and, during the run/walk periods, respond to it. Need to work at a lower RPE level for the run part? That's OK. Need to walk for longer? That's OK, too. Aim to cover 15 minutes your way.

# WEEK 3

## WARM-UP
5-minute walk with purpose (RPE 2/amber) followed by mobility work.

### RUN 1

**RUN TO FEEL**

A 15–20-minute session.

Run this session as you feel for 15–20 minutes. The effort you are looking to be at is RPE 3–4/green.

Start with a 2:2 walk/run and stay at that or, if you feel good, try a 2:1.

Still feeling good? How might it feel to keep a consistent, comfortable RPE 4/green jog?

### COOL-DOWN

**WALK COOL-DOWN**
(RPE 1/amber) for 5 minutes followed by gentle stretching.

### RUN 2

**RUN TO FEEL**

A 10–15-minute session.

No instructions other than to move your body for between 10 and 15 minutes. Do it your way but aim to keep to that RPE 3–4/green effort level.

## NOTES

**RUN 1**
How does it feel to have a choice on how you move? Remember, your body will tell you what it needs. Listen to those RPE cues we talked about in chapter 5 (*see* p. 70). This run is about mixing it up, but only if you want to.

**RUN 2**
What is your body telling you? Are you tired? Are you energised? Tune in and respond to that.

# WEEK 4

## WARM-UP
5-minute walk with purpose/gentle jog (RPE 2/amber–green).
Mix it up depending on how you feel! Follow it with mobility work.

### RUN 1

**MOUND OF OPPORTUNITY**

Find a gentle hill or incline. When you are at the bottom, remember all that I discussed with you in chapter 7 (see pp. 98–105).

You are going to run up this incline/hill either as a run/walk starting at 10 seconds up (RPE 4–5/green–red) and then you are going to turn around and walk back (RPE 1–2/amber) taking the recovery time that you need before you start ascending the hill again. Each time you run/walk or run up the hill you will increase the time by 5 seconds (10, 15, 20, 25, etc.). The aim is that you are working at a level that will feel uncomfortable on the uphill and then you will be recovering on the downhill to get your breath back – ready to turn around, look up and go again.

Repeat reps up and down for 15 minutes. Keep track of how many you do in this time, too.

### COOL-DOWN

Gentle jog for 5–10 minutes (RPE 2) or 2:2 run/walk for 5–10 minutes followed by stretching.

### RUN 2

**RUN TO FEEL**
A 15-minute session.
Do this run as feels right for you. This can be a gentle run (RPE 3–4/green), a run walk (2:2 or 2:1 of what feels right) or a combination of it all.
Do what feels right.

## NOTES

**RUN 1**
Ensure you are taking enough time to recover on the downhill. There is no time attributed to this. Your recovery and readiness to go again uphill is based on how you feel.

**RUN 2**
How are you feeling after that hill session? Tune into your body and do what feels right on this run.

# WEEK 5

### WARM-UP
5-minute walk with purpose/jog (RPE 2/amber) as you feel, leading into mobility work.

## RUN 1

### RUN TO FEEL
A 25-minute session.

Today you are going to be increasing the *time on your feet* during this – the main part – of the run session.

I want you to move for up to 25 minutes at RPE 4/green.

I'd like you to start off at a gentle jog. Can you hold a conversation as the minutes roll by? If not, slow down and use a 3:2, 2:2 or 2:1 run/walk protocol until you feel ready to run for longer.

## COOL-DOWN

### WALK COOL-DOWN
Gentle jog for 5–10 minutes (RPE 2–3/amber–green) or jog/walk or just walk. Stretch.

## RUN 2

### FARTLEK
Run to feel during the majority of this session by running or doing a walk/run (RPE 3/green).

At six points in this run – when you choose to do it – I want you to go a bit faster (RPE 5–6/red) for 30 seconds.

Always give yourself time to recover after each speedier bit (you might choose to walk for 1–2 minutes and then take it back to a gentle jog). It's your call.

### NOTES

**RUN 1**
We are increasing that endurance this week, on this run. This is the longest you will have run for. Go you!

**RUN 2**
This week is a challenging one. How do you feel? What's happening with your hormone levels?

Remember, it all feeds into how you will perform on the run.

# WEEK 6

## WARM-UP
10-minute walk with purpose/gentle jog (RPE 2/amber) as you feel, leading into mobility work.

### RUN 1

**EFFORT PLAY**

A 25-minute session.

Over the course of this run I want you to play with your effort via walking, very comfortable running and faster running.

What does it feel like moving from RPE 3/green through the elevated effort levels to RPE 6/red? What are your body and mind telling you?

### COOL-DOWN

**WALK COOL-DOWN**

Gentle jog or run/walk for 5 minutes (RPE 2/amber) followed by stretching.

### RUN 2

**RUN TO FEEL**

A 20-minute session.

A really gentle run, jog or walk as appropriate for how you are feeling this week.

Aim to be out for 20 minutes.

## NOTES

**RUN 1**
How easy do you find it to speed up? To slow down? To find that comfortable forever pace?

**RUN 2**
The sessions are starting to build consistency and time on feet but this run is really about being present in your body. How are you feeling, mentally, physically? Do what feels right for you.

# WEEK 7

## WARM-UP
10-minute walk with purpose/gentle jog (RPE 2–3/amber–green) as you feel, leading into mobility work.

### RUN 1

**RUN TO FEEL**

A 30-minute session.

Run or run/walk as you feel. Remember to keep your effort level moderate (RPE 3/green) and start really gently.

### COOL-DOWN

**WALK COOL-DOWN**

Gentle jog or run/walk for 5–10 minutes (RPE 2/amber) followed by stretching.

### RUN 2

**RUN TO FEEL**

Mound of opportunity.

Remember that gentle hill or incline that I asked you to find in week 4? I want you to go there again.

Remember my hill-running tips (see pp. 98–105)!

You are going up this incline/hill as a run, taking walk breaks on the uphill section only if you need them. You are going to go up for 30 seconds (RPE 5–6/red) and then you are going to turn around and walk back down (RPE 2/amber).

Remember, the aim of this session is that you are working at a level that will feel uncomfortable on the uphill and you will be recovering on the down – to get your breath back – ready to eventually turn around, look up and go again.

Please repeat 6 times.

## NOTES

**RUN 1**
We are building up that time on your feet again, little by little. Think back to week 1 – look how far you have already come!

**RUN 2**
How did it feel on this hill three weeks on? If harder, why? If easier, why?!

# WEEK 8

## WARM-UP
10-minute walk with purpose/gentle jog (RPE 2/amber) as you feel, leading into mobility work.

### RUN 1

**OUT AND BACK**

A 10-minute session.

You get to choose the effort level you want to work to on this one. If you want to, keep it at RPE 4/green, ensuring you are comfortable all the way, then do that.

Or maybe you want to work a bit harder (RPE 5–6/red) for the duration of the run. If so, try that. You can always come back down in effort if it feels like too much.

You are in control.

### COOL-DOWN

**WALK COOL-DOWN**

10-minute gentle jog (RPE 2–3) followed by stretching.

### RUN 2

**GRATITUDE RUN**

A 20-minute session.

I want you to do a gentle run or run/walk (RPE 3/green) during this run.

Every 5 minutes I want you to think about something or someone you are grateful for. If it's to do with the process of learning to run, great. If not, it doesn't matter. Be present and give yourself gratitude for being on this journey.

## NOTES

**RUN 1**
You are in control! Think back to week 2. Can you remember how far you got in either 5 or 7 minutes? Did you make a note of it? Where did you get to today?! And how did you feel?

**RUN 2**
I am grateful for you and to you for being on week 8 of this journey.

# WEEK 9

### WARM-UP
10-minute walk with purpose/gentle jog (RPE 2/amber) as you feel, leading into mobility work.

## RUN 1

**EFFORT PLAY**

A 30-minute session.

Over the course of this run I want you to play with your effort via walking, very comfortable running and faster running.

What does it feel like moving from RPE 2/amber through the elevated effort levels to RPE 6/red? What are your body and mind telling you?

Move up and down through the levels as you *feel*.

### COOL-DOWN

10-minute easy run (RPE 2–3) followed by stretching.

## RUN 2

**RUN TO FEEL**

A 25-minute session.

I want you to run to feel. You are almost there! This is your last session before your 5K 'graduation run'. Keep this run very gentle (RPE 3/green). It should feel super comfortable. If it doesn't then slow it down to a run/walk.

### NOTES

**RUN 1**
How easy do you find it to speed up? To slow down? To find that comfortable forever pace?

**RUN 2**
I want you to remember that I am so proud of all you have done. You are a superstar!

# WEEK 10

## WARM-UP

10-minute walk with purpose/gentle jog (RPE 2/amber) as you feel, leading into mobility work.

### RUN 1

**GRADUATION RUN!**

Pick a 5K run – a Parkrun would be perfect – and move your body around the route by running or run/walking in a way that feels good for you.

Some women like the idea of being with other people for this graduation run, while others want to create a route themselves and do it solo.

Do the 5K your way!

The key thing is that you do the 5K run and celebrate your 10-week journey.

### COOL-DOWN

5-minute gentle walk/jog (RPE 2/amber) followed by stretching . . . AND CAKE!

### RUN 2

Not this week.

## NOTES

You did it!

I am so proud of you!

## 4 The cool-down

Just as the warm-up is important, so is your cool-down. Taking time – and in this plan I advise spending 5–10 minutes on cooling down – will help your wonderful body to transition from higher-intensity movement to a resting state. Taking time to cool down by doing a low-RPE run or walk helps you by:

- **Stopping you feeling dizzy** – Your heart will have been beating faster than it is maybe used to, so you need to bring it back down gradually. Stopping running suddenly can make blood pool in your legs, which will make you feel dizzy.
- **Making you less sore** – Every time you are running you are creating tiny tears in your muscles. A gentle cool-down will help to flush out lactic acid effectively, which will reduce post-run soreness and stiffness.
- **Getting you into relax mode more quickly** – A cool-down will reduce your heart rate and breathing rate gradually. This will help your body recover faster and your nervous system to shift from 'work' to 'relax' mode and start sending the signal for tissues to begin to heal.

## 5 Stretching

Don't worry, you're almost there. But don't forget this bit. Taking some time to stretch after your run is a really important part of your recovery and will help to prevent injuries, too. You don't need to spend ages stretching, as I know how, post run, life starts to creep into your mind and you need to get in that shower and back to kids, work, partner, the dog, etc. That's why below I have included only what I believe to be essential stretches for new runners.

But why stretch, you might ask? Here are some very good reasons:

- Over time, regular stretching will improve your flexibility, which will make it easier for you to maintain good running form and prevent injuries.

- You'll have a greater range of motion in places like your hips and hamstrings – essential for running.
- If your muscles aren't stretched out after a run, they can become tight and prone to cramping. The stretches below will help to lengthen the muscles, improving how elastic they are and reducing cramps and stiffness, especially in your legs.
- Tight muscles can affect your posture and body alignment, which can lead to imbalances and discomfort over time. Practising stretching will open up tight areas (like your hips) and restore muscle balance, which will improve your posture and overall movement.
- It'll reduce your risk of injuries by maintaining joint health and reducing the chances of muscle strains and sprains.
- It'll allow you to cool down mentally, too, by helping you focus on movement and breathing in readiness for a more relaxed state of being.

## The stretches

Below I have shared a number of static stretches. These can be done outside, once you have finished your cool-down, or inside where it might be warmer. It doesn't matter where you do them, just that they are done.

## CALF STRETCH

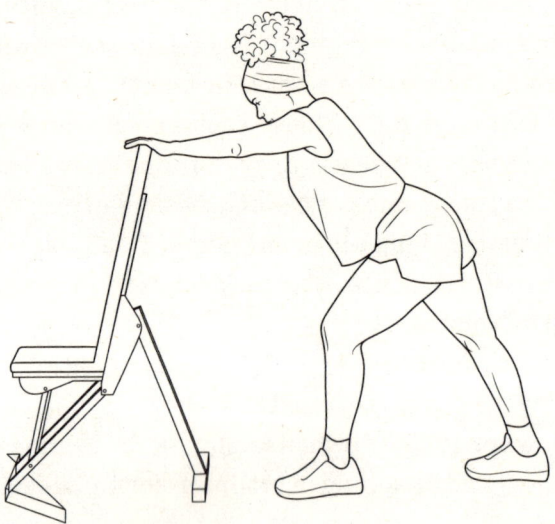

Place both hands on a wall, sturdy surface, or the back of a chair. You will be facing the thing you are leaning on. Engage your core and step one foot back, keeping your heel on the ground, then bend your front knee. Press your hips forwards, keeping that heel on the floor and feel the stretch in the calf – that's the muscle in your lower leg, above the ankle. Hold for 20–30 seconds, then go back to the starting position and repeat on the other side.

## STANDING QUAD STRETCH

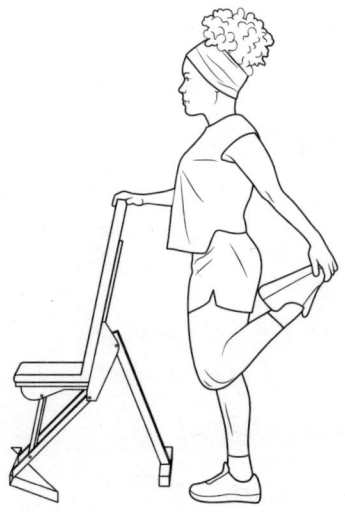

Stand tall and, if you need to, hold onto a wall or a chair for balance, keeping your core engaged. Now bend your right leg behind you and, if you can, take hold of your right ankle with your right hand. If you can't reach your ankle, hold your trainer at the back of the top of the heel. Now gently pull your right foot towards your bum. Try to keep your knees close together and in line with each other. Hold for 20–30 seconds, then release and repeat the stretch on the opposite leg. You should feel a slight pull in the front of the bent leg, between your knee and hip.

## HAMSTRING STRETCH

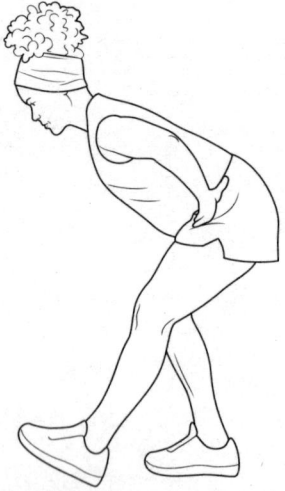

Stand tall. Keeping your core engaged, extend one leg out straight, resting your heel on the ground with your toes pointing up. Bend yourself forwards at the hips (not your back), keeping your back straight (try not to let it curve). Rest your hands on your hips. You should feel a slight pull in the back of the leg that is straight – between the back of the knee and the bum. Hold for 20–30 seconds, then release and repeat on the opposite leg.

## UPPER BACK STRETCH

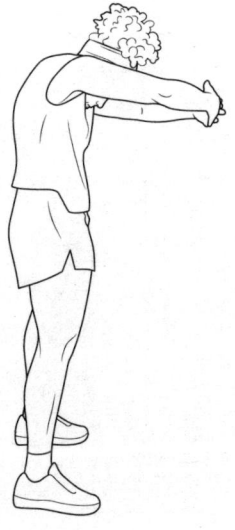

Stand tall, engage the core and clasp your hands together in front of you. Now round your upper back, pressing your hands forwards and tucking in your chin. Really focus on rounding that upper back (I like to imagine I am trying to sprout wings). Hold for 20–30 seconds, then release.

## CHEST STRETCH

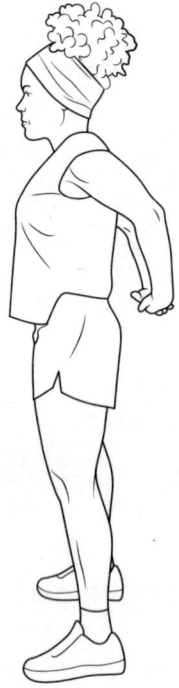

Stand tall, shoulders relaxed, and engage the core. Clasp your hands behind your back. Now straighten your arms and gently lift them away from your body, standing tall, while opening your chest. Hold for 20–30 seconds, then release.

**Don't forget to breathe!**
Even though you are at the end of your run practice, I don't want you to forget to breathe. I see this in a lot of women, especially those new to stretching. They are so focused on holding the position that they start holding their breath, too. I need you to keep feeding oxygen into the body in order to fuel the movement. You are looking to breathe very steadily, in for two and out for two. Take big, deep breaths to encourage muscle release and flush out any remaining lactic acid. Close your eyes, if you so wish. Post-run stretching can be a really great way to recentre yourself ready for whatever may come next in your life.

CHAPTER 14

# A final message from me . . .

So, what else is there to say that has not already been said? You have all the information you need from me, from experts and from the amazing women who have shared their stories and their tips with you. I believe in you and think that you are now ready to start where you are. I wish I could be there with you but know that I am in spirit! Please do share your running journey with me via social media. I'd like to consider myself as part of your virtual community and, who knows, one day we might get to run together in person.

    If there was one piece of final advice I could give you it would be to keep your WHY close by. What I mean is always remember why you started. Why you are doing this. Because there will be hard times when you need to remember that why. It's the thing that will keep you going. For me, as you know, it was to be a better mum. To be mentally well. And now, I run to show others that they can too, if only they dare to try. We can all do hard things. And, for us women runners, that hard thing starts with the decision to try.

    I can't wait to see you out there!

# And from the women . . .

'Just do it! Don't worry about what others think.'

'It doesn't matter what you look like, you can run! Have confidence in yourself, as you can do it.'

'Stick with it. Keep going, as the benefits are life-changing!'

'Take it as slowly as you need to, so that you can chat and run. A 5K, is a 5K , is a 5K.'

'Take your time. It is a slow process and it's not linear. Enjoy all the emotions of learning how to run.'

'Keep at it! You will get better and enjoy it.'

'Don't be afraid to start, it could change your life.'

# References

## Chapter 1
'Since 2023, at least 25 countries have introduced social prescribing': https://socialprescribingacademy.org.uk/media/thtjrirn/social-prescribing-around-the-world-2024.pdf

## Chapter 2
'There's a ton of research out there that shows that men': www.tandfonline.com/doi/full/10.1080/21520704.2020.1826615

'When they are not training or racing, they try *not* to stand up.': Laura Kenny

'Never stand when you can sit, never sit when you can lie down.': Chris Hoy, https://www.belfasttelegraph.co.uk/sport/columnists/billy-on-the-box/billy-on-the-box-chris-hoy-switches-gears-and-machines-for-his-new-sporting-challenge/35126698.html

'Only 6 per cent of sports-related research is conducted on female only participants': Cowley *et al.*, 202; https://researchportal.northumbria.ac.uk/en/publications/invisible-sportswomen-the-sex-data-gap-in-sport-and-exercise-scie

'The change model is called the Transtheoretical Model of Behaviour': Prochaska, J. O., DiClemente, C. C. and Norcross, J. C., 'In search of the structure of change'. In Y. Klar, J. D. Fisher, J. M. Chinsky and A. Nadler (Eds.), *Self-change: Social psychological and clinical perspectives* (New York: Springer Verlag, 1992) pp. 87–114.

'A report by ASICS called "Closing the Gender Exercise Gap"': www.asics.com/us/en-us/mk/move-her-mind/report

## Chapter 3
'Around 30–35 per cent of new runners': pubmed.ncbi.nlm.nih.gov/30071170/

'Studies show that one of the reasons runners tend to get injured': https://pmc.ncbi.nlm.nih.gov/articles/PMC4338213/

## Chapter 4
'The estimated value of the global running gear market by 2033 is $66.9 billion': https://vocal.media/journal/running-gear-market-an-in-depth-analysis

'The average breast size in the UK is 36DD': https://www.healthline.com/health/average-breast-size

'Consequences of not wearing a sports bra': www.runandbecome.com/running-product-advice/why-wear-a-sports-bra-when-running#:~:text=The%20breast%20is%20only%20supported,when%20exercising%2C%20especially%20when%20running.

'In 2022, an estimated 2.3 million women were diagnosed with breast cancer worldwide': https://www.who.int/news-room/fact-sheets/detail/breast-cancer#:~:text=In%202022%2C%20there%20were%202.3,use%20and%20postmenopausal%20hormone%20therapy.

'Gen Z report as preferring baggy clothing, whereas Millennials prefer tight clothing': https://www.bbc.com/culture/article/20240426-cargo-pants-v-skinny-jeans-gen-z-and-millennials-fight-it-out

'A "Year In Sport" report by Strava in 2025': https://press.strava.com/articles/strava-releases-annual-year-in-sport-trend

## Chapter 5

'64.5 per cent of participants dropped out, with 74.6 per cent dropping out before the halfway point': pmc.ncbi.nlm.nih.gov/articles/PMC10487403/

## Chapter 6

'research shows that the knee joint alone': https://pubmed.ncbi.nlm.nih.gov/23377837/

## Chapter 8

'A 2024 survey by the University of Manchester': www.manchester.ac.uk/about/news/majority-of-women-experience-abuse-while-running/

'An Our Streets Now survey': www.ourstreetsnow.org/case-studies-1/blog-post-title-three-3b7wa

'the UK Athletics RunTogether website is a resource to use': runtogether.co.uk

'I [. . .] use a service called what3words': www.what3words.com

'95 per cent of women respondents said that they didn't report the abuse they'd encountered': www.manchester.ac.uk/about/news/majority-of-women-experience-abuse-while-running/

'in the UK it is illegal for any member of the public to carry a lethal or non-lethal self-defence weapon': brittontime.com/2021/10/22/everything-you-need-to-know-about-self-defence-law-in-the-uk/

'If you are abused, *please* tell someone': www.ourstreetsnow.org/case-studies-1/blog-post-title-three-3b7wa

'An Adidas survey found that 92 per cent of 4,500 women': news.adidas.com/running/new-adidas-study-finds-92--of-women-are-concerned-for-their-safety-when-they-go-for-a-run/s/c318f69e-7575-4ced-bbf3-9db6d2ab1642

## Chapter 9

'In 2022, the UK charity Women in Sport (WIS) surveyed 4,000 teenage girls': https://womeninsport.org/resource/reframing-sport-for-teenage-girls-tackling-teenage-disengagement/

'The WIS survey found that 59 per cent of teenage girls': https://womeninsport.org/resource/reframing-sport-for-teenage-girls-tackling-teenage-disengagement/

'There is good, robust evidence to show that [...] using starflower oil can be helpful': https://www.simplysupplements.co.uk/healthylife/women-and-health/starflower-oil-benefits-for-womens-health#:~:text=One%20study%20found%20that%20daily%20supplementation%20with,of%2040%25)%20when%20compared%20to%20a%20placebo.&text=One%20placebo%2Dcontrolled%20trial%20found%20that%20daily%20supplementation,67%25%20respectively%20when%20compared%20to%20a%20placebo.

'Research shows that a woman's basal metabolic rate': https://pubmed.ncbi.nlm.nih.gov/7124662/

## Chapter 10

Research shows that many women have had success in using supplements and herbal remedies to manage specific symptoms, and potential deficiencies, caused by menopause such as insomnia, mood regulation, anxiety, bone strength etc. These supplement and remedies include but not limited to: https://www.cochranelibrary.com/cdsr/doi/10.1002/14651858.CD007244.pub2/full

'Bovine collagen is the most supported with scientific studies': https://pmc.ncbi.nlm.nih.gov/articles/PMC8620403/

'Studies show that perimenopausal women who have used these herbal remedies': https://www.naturesbest.co.uk/our-blog/the-menopause/should-i-be-taking-evening-primrose-oil-for-menopause/

'If you do not moisturise your vagina then it can be prone to irritation and tearing': bssm.org.uk/wp-content/uploads/2024/03/BSSM-Position-statement-for-management-of-genitourinary-syndrome-of-the-menopause-GSM.pdf

'There are websites that allow you to do your own simple bone assessment': www.fraxplus.org

'vitamin D supplementation is a must in the autumn and winter months': www.nhs.uk/conditions/vitamins-and-minerals/vitamin-d/

## Chapter 12

Renee McGregor, *Fuel For Thought* (Vertebrate Publishing Ltd, 2025)

'Science shows that our bodies have enough stored energy to keep moving well for up to 90 minutes': https://pmc.ncbi.nlm.nih.gov/articles/PMC3302369/

'A market that is estimated to be worth $94 billion by 2033': https://straitsresearch.com/report/sports-nutrition-market

Anita Bean, *The Runner's Cookbook* (Bloomsbury, 2017)

Do you know how much water we as women are supposed to consume a day? Well, for the average woman (hey, who are you calling average!) it's 6–8 cups or glasses a day: https://www.nhs.uk/live-well/eat-well/food-guidelines-and-food-labels/water-drinks-nutrition/ https://www.nutrition.org.uk/nutritional-information/hydration/

Are you a lover of cow's milk? If so, read on! https://pubmed.ncbi.nlm.nih.gov/30379113/

# Bibliography

Bean, Anita, *The Runner's Cookbook*, (Bloomsbury, 2017)

Kirk-Odenumbi, Emma, *Find Your Pace: How running changed my life and how it can change yours too*, (Bluebird, 2026)

McGregor, Renee, *Training Food: Get the fuel you need to achieve your goals*, (Nourish Books, 2015)

McGregor, Renee, *More Fuel You: Understanding your body and how to fuel your adventures*, (Vertebrate Publishing Ltd., 2022)

McGregor, Renee, *Fuel for Thought: A practical guide for fuelling your adventures*, (Vertebrate Publishing Ltd, 2025)

Sims, Stacy, T., *Roar: Match your food and fitness to your unique female physiology for optimum performance, gut health and a strong body for life*, (Harmony/Rodale, 2016)

# Acknowledgements

To every woman who has ever doubted she could be a runner, this book is for you.

Writing *Start Where You Are* has been a journey of reflection, gratitude and joy for me. This book is as much the product of community as it is my voice.

I absolutely could not have brought it into being without so many wonderful people who believe in me and the message I aim to convey within these pages. It really does take a village!

First and foremost, to my family – my husband, my four children and my three grandchildren. Thank you for your unconditional love for me even when I get your names mixed up (perimenopause!) Thanks also for your patience in me when I am so engrossed in a task that I forget to look up and for your endless support of my life adventures. You give me the strength to lace up, to write and to keep showing up, even on the days it feels really hard. You are my constant reminder of why movement matters.

To the incredible women both past and present of *Stroud Mums on the Run* – thank you for trusting me as your coach over the years, for every laugh, every tear and every mile you've allowed me to lead you on. You taught me what community truly means and why no woman should ever feel left behind.

To my *Black Trail Runners* family – thank you for standing alongside me in the work of representation, access and belonging for *all* in the running space. You remind me every day that change happens when we dare to show up.

To the many women who shared their stories so honestly with me within these pages, your courage and vulnerability make this book what it is. Thank you for reminding the people reading this book that running isn't about perfection, it's about persistence and heart.

To each and every expert who so generously shared their wisdom, your insights have brought authority, evidence and compassion to these chapters. I am eternally grateful to you for the work you do.

To my brilliant agent, Sarah Such, for your steadfast belief in this book and constant guidance. And to Charlotte, Sarah S and everyone at Bloomsbury Sport – thank you for believing in the concept of this book, in me as an author and ensuring this book reaches the women who need it most.

And finally, to you, my reader. Words cannot express my gratitude for you choosing to Start Where You Are. My measure of success will be in witnessing – either via social media or in person – your journey. Keep me updated! And always remember, 'You can do hard things!'

Take the first step, breathe deeply and keep going. I'm right beside you.

# Index

abdominal strength   191
abuse
   physical   116–17
   verbal   116
amino acids   201
anaemia   154
arm holders   60
arm movement   33–4, 99, 103, 104
arm sleeves   56
author's story   6–12, 196–7

backpacks   59–60
bags   57–60
barriers to running   15–16, 19, 23
basal metabolic rate   136
beginner running behaviour, five
      stages   20–2
belts, running   59
Black Girls Do Run UK   20, 117
body image   162
bone health   137, 159, 161
'bonking'   84
BORG Effort Scale and traffic-light
      system   67–8
Bound, Mel   109, 110
bowel urgency   158, 209–10
bras, sports   47–52, 58
breathing   27, 30–2, 82, 100, 243
buddies/friends, running   109–10, 146
bum bags/fanny packs   58–9

cadence, running   36–7, 98
carbohydrates   136–7, 148, 197–9,
      208, 210
catcalling/verbal abuse   116
chafe management   60–2
childbirth and female runners   190–1
chunking a run   84–5
clothing   62
   bags   57–60
   chafe management   60–2
   layering   56, 148
   managing body temperature   148
   nice-to-haves   55–6
   reflective clothing/hi vis   111
   second-hand items   56–7
   sports bras   47–52, 58
   technical clothing   53–5

tight v baggy   53–4
trainers   40–6, 57
co-ordination   161
collagen   155–6
consistency, effort   101
core engagement   34–6, 103
Couch to 5K programmes   64, 143–4,
      153
   author's   213–14, 243
      1. the warm-up   214–15
      2. mobility exercises   215–21
      3. the sessions
         effort play   224
         fartlek   224
         gratitude run   224
         mounds of opportunity/hill
            runs   224
         out and back   223–4
         rate of perceived exertion
            (RPE)   222
         run to feel   223
         walk with purpose   223
         Week 1   226
         Week 2   227
         Week 3   228
         Week 4   229
         Week 5   230
         Week 6   231
         Week 7   232
         Week 8   233
         Week 9   234
         Week 10   235
      4. the cool down   236
      5. stretching   236–42

dark, running in the   108–11
dehydration, signs of   206–7
delayed onset muscle soreness
      (DOMS)   166, 201, 211
depression   9
diaphragmatic (belly) breathing   31–2
downhill running   103

electrolytes   202, 207
elite athletes   13–14, 25–6, 79
elitist attitudes to running   16–18
endorphins   70, 130
endurance, increased   161

energy leakage  34
exercises
    form explained  179
    glute/bum focused  192–3
    hip airplane  193
    jargon buster  166
    pelvic floor exercises  158, 192
    strength and conditioning  168, 213
        core  177
            dead bug  180
            half plank  178
            oblique twist  181
        lower body
            slouch  171–2
            spit squats  170
            squats  169
        plyometrics/jumping  182
            forward jumps  185
            jump squat  183
            skipping  186
            speed skater  184
        routine/session structure  186–8
        upper body  172
            modified push-ups  174
            single-arm dumbbell row  176
            standing dumbbell arm swing  175
            wall push-ups  173
    stretches  236–7
        calf stretch  238
        chest stretch  242
        hamstring stretch  240
        standing quad stretch  239
        upper back stretch  241
    warm-up  214–15
        ankle rotations  221
        arm circles  218
        butt kicks  96
        heel-to-toe walks  97
        high knees  95
        leg swings  93
        neck rotations  216
        neck tilts  217
        squats  220
        standing hip circles  219
        walking lunges with torso twist  94

failure, fear of  19
fartlek  224
fat-burning zone  72–3
fatigue, perimenopause and  144–6
fatigue, post-run  83–4

fitness tracking apps  115
flexibility  162, 215
food and drink  195–7
    avoiding tummy troubles  209–10
    carbohydrates  136–7, 148, 197–9, 208, 210
    cow's milk  205
    eating enough/nourishing  199–200, 208–9
    electrolytes  202, 207
    hydration  150, 206–7
    iron-rich foods  155
    menstrual cycle  136–7
    portion sizes  198
    protein  150, 205–6
    recovery fuelling  201
    snacks on the run  73, 202–4
    sports nutrition market  204–5
    weight gain  151–2
    when to eat  200
foot strike  37–8
form/technique, running  25–6, 90
    1. posture  28–30
    2. breathing  30–2
    3. arm movement  33–4
    4. core engagement  34–6
    5. stride length and cadence  36–7
    6. foot strike  37–8
    downhill running  103–4
    hill running  90, 98–102
    'teeth and tits'  28
friends, running with  109–10, 146

gait, running  42
    analysis  43
Galloway, Jeff  86
gaze direction  99
gender bias in sports science  18, 65–6
Gerardi, Hillary  79
gloves  56
glutes (bum muscles)  190
GPS trackers  114
gymnasiums  163–4

headbands and buffs  55–6
headphones  112
heart rate  31, 72, 81–2, 133–4, 215
    hear rate variance (HRV)  134–5
    resting heart rate (RHR)  134
heel strike  37–8, 100
high-intensity interval training (HIIT)  90

hill running 87–9, 104–5, 224
  benefits 90–1
  downhill 103–4
  technique for beginners 99–102
  warm-up 92–7
hormone levels 65, 71, 126, 130, 137, 142–3, 147–8, 149, 155, 156–7
  *see also* menstrual cycle
hormone replacement therapy (HRT) 156–7
hot flashes 147–8
Hoy, Sir Chris 14
hybrid shoes 46
hydration 150, 206–7

injuries 27, 36, 38, 39, 83, 128, 161, 188, 215
iron levels 153–5, 211

jackets 55
joint pain 142–3

Kegel exercises 192
Kenny, Dame Laura 13–14
Kipchoge, Eliud 26
Kirk-Odunubi, Emma 26, 36, 43
KT tape 61

leakage, urinary 158, 191–2
leggings 54
Lingam-Willgoss, Dr Candice 20
lost, getting 113–14

Magness, Steve 82
male bias, sports research 18, 65–6, 78
mantras, empowering 24
McGregor, Renee 124, 134, 135, 136, 137, 153–4, 201, 208–9, 211
menopause and perimenopause 138, 159
  10 minute goals 145
  body temperature 147
  bone health 159
  dietary supplements 153–6
  fatigue 144–6
  flooding 138–9, 155
  hormone replacement therapy (HRT) 156–7
  joint pain 142–3
  mindful running 145–6
  'nanna naps' 146
  and running 141–3
  running with friends 146
  symptoms 139–40, 141–3
  tendonitis 149–51
  vaginal health 158
  weight gain 151–2
menstrual cycle
  bloating and discomfort 130–1
  fatigue and low energy 130
  follicular phase and running 127
  food and drink 136
  heart rate 133–5
  hormone fatigue 126
  keeping track 126
  luteal phase and running 128–9
  managing flows and leaks 131–2
  managing symptoms 131, 135–6
  menstrual phase and running 127
  missed periods 137
  ovulatory phase and running 128
  pain and cramps 129
  periods and sport 122–4
  phases overview 125
  *see also* menopause and perimenopause
mental health 70
  mental fatigue 144–5
mindfulness 145–6
mindset, runner's 13
Munro, Dr Cath 141–3, 153–4, 157, 158
muscle building and muscle mass 161–7
  *see also* exercises; strength and conditioning training

'nanna naps' 146
networks, female runner 109–10
neutral pronation 42
nighttime running 108–11

oestrogen 125, 128, 137, 142, 147, 149, 152, 158
Olympic Games 78
osteoporosis 159
overpronation 42
overthinking 70
overtraining 214
oxygen levels 90, 161

pace, running
  hormone levels 65
  listening to your body/RPE training 63–4, 67–75
  running too fast 63, 76–7
  training programmes and apps 64–5
  *see also* walking breaks

parkruns  10
Parkwalk event  80
pelvic floor  191–2
   exercises  158, 192–3
perimenopause *see* menopause and perimenopause
periods and running  122–4, 129–33, 155
   *see also* menopause and perimenopause; menstrual cycle
periods, missed  137
phones  58, 112, 135
physical abuse  116–17
physiotherapists  151, 189, 194
plyometric strength  90
poo, needing a  209–10
postnatal depression  9
posture, running  28–30
pregnancy and childbirth  190–1
progesterone  125, 129, 155
protein  150, 201

racial inclusivity  107–8
Radcliffe, Paula  26
rate of perceived exertion (RPE) training  64, 67
   Borg Effort Scale and traffic-light system  67–70, 74–5, 222–3
   cues
      breathing and exertion  70–1
      energy requirements  72–3
      heart rate  72
      listen to your muscles  72
      mental and emotional effort  73
      reading the cues  73–4
      sweat rate  71–2
      temperature  71–2
Raynaud's syndrome  56
reasons to start running  6, 14–15
recovery and rest  102, 151, 152–3, 201
   *see also* walking breaks
reflective clothing  111
relative energy deficiency in sport (REDS)  208
reporting abuse  116, 118–19
resilience, mental  107–8
resting  151
road shoes  45–6
route variation  115
run analysts  43
'runner' stereotype  16

safety matters  23, 58, 106–7, 120–1
   getting lost  113–14
   online safety  115
   physical abuse  117–18
   racial abuse  119–20
   route variation  115
   running alone  111–14
   running in the dark  108–11
   tracking apps and GPS  113, 114
   verbal abuse  116
self-defence  118
shoes, running  40–6, 57
shorts and skorts  54
Sims, Dr Stacy  18, 190–1
sleep  146
snacks on the run  73, 202–4
social prescribing  9
socks  55
speed, running  63, 76–7
   and weight  208–9
sports clothing industry  16–17
sports-related research, male bias  18, 65–6, 78
starflower oil  135–6
steps per minute (SPM)  98–9
stereotype, 'runner'  16, 19
strength and conditioning training  160–1, 213
   20 minute goal  166–7
   barriers to  162–3
   benefits of  161–2
   delayed onset muscle soreness (DOMS)  166
   exercises  168, 169–88
   how should it feel?  165–6
   increased running resilience  165
   patience and results  167
   trainers  168
   *see also* exercises
stress hormones  130, 147
stretching  236–42
stride length and cadence  36–7, 98
sunglasses  56
supination  42
supplements, dietary  136, 153–6, 211
sweating  71, 131
   salty  202
swelling feet  44–5

taping  61–2
Taylor-Swaine, Bethan  65–6
technique, running *see* form/technique, running

temperature, body   71–2, 147–8
tendonitis/tendon niggles   149–51, 188–90
terrain, types of   45–6
testosterone   137, 164
thermoregulation   147–8
This Girl Can campaign   18
This Woman Runs (TWR)   109
Thompson, Tasha   20, 117–18
tops, running   54–5
torches, head and chest   110–11
tracking apps   113
trail shoes   45–6
trainers
   foot size and width   43–4
   running gait   42–3
   second-hand   57
   strength and conditioning training   168
   sustainable running   46
   tendonitis   150
   what terrain?   45–6
training plans and apps   64–5
Transtheoretical Model of Behaviour   20–1
tummy troubles   209–10

underpronation   42
urinary/bowel urgency   158, 209–10

vaginal health   158
verbal abuse   116
visualisation technique, hill run   99
vitamin and mineral supplements   153–6, 211
$VO_2$ max   90

walking breaks   76–80
   to chunk/cut up the run   84–5
   hill running   100–1, 102
   improving form and breathing   82
   increasing overall running session time   83
   increasing the joy   85
   keeping it fun   86
   keeping it social   85
   maintaining comfortable heart rate   81–2
   recover on the move   82
   reducing post run fatigue   83–4
   reducing risk of injury   83
   support running progression   80–1
Wallace, Keri   101, 103
warm-up exercises   93–7, 150, 214–15
   for mobility   215–21
weight, body   151–2, 207–9

zone   2/aerobic heart rate   81–2